MANAGEMENT OF HEART FAILURE

by

Jay N. Cohn, M.D.

Professor of Medicine
Head, Cardiovascular Division
University of Minnesota Medical School
Minneapolis, MN

Spencer H. Kubo, M.D.

Assistant Professor of Medicine
Medical Director,
Heart Failure/Heart Transplantation Program
Cardiovascular Division
University of Minnesota Medical School
Minneapolis, MN

**Essential Medical
Information Systems, Inc.**
Durant, Oklahoma

Essential Medical
Information Systems, Inc.
P.O. Box 1607
Durant, OK 74702

To order, please call:

Independent Distributor:
Education and Technology Company
(800) 344-7686
Order #7-7-8

FIRST EDITION

ISBN: 0-929240-17-0

Published in the United States 1991

Printed in the United States of America

Center Index Texts Published by

Essential Medical Information Systems, Inc.:

Management of Hypertension-3rd Ed. — Kaplan

Estrogen Replacement Therapy-2nd Ed. — Gambrell

Contraceptive Sterilization — Moss

Hormonal Contraception: Pills, Injections & Implants — Goldzieher

Breastfeeding: A Problem-Solving Manual-2nd Ed. — Johnson, Carroll & Saunders

Diagnosing and Managing Chemical Dependency — Beasley

Menopause: Clinical Concepts — London & Chihal

Premenstrual Syndrome-2nd Ed. — Chihal

Management of Diabetes Mellitus — Schwartz

Children With Special Needs-2nd Ed. — Bradway & Block

Assessment and Management of the Suicidal Adolescent — Clayton

Infertility: A Clinician's Manual — Cohen

Management of Lipid Disorders — Leaf

Anesthesia Guide — Jerome

Mid-Life Sexuality: Enrichment and Problem Solving — Semmens

Estrogen Replacement Therapy User Guide — Gambrell

Hyptertension Treatment: User Guide — Kaplan

Request Catalog for complete list of center index texts.

TABLE OF CONTENTS

General Information
Definitions of Cardiac Failure 8
Causes of Cardiac Failure
and Cardiomyopathy 12
Signs and Symptoms
Clinical Signs and Symptoms 20
Pathophysiology
Starling Curve and Impedance/
Outflow Resistance 24
Vicious Cycle of Heart Failure 28
Salt and Water Reabsorption 30
Exercise Intolerance 32
Precipitating Causes of CHF/Survival 36
Laboratory Assessment
Electrocardiogram/Chest X-Ray 40
Echocardiogram/Doppler/Nuclear
Heart Scan 44
Cardiac Catheterization 48
Endomyocardial Biopsy 52
Exercise Testing 56
Diuretics
Dietary Sodium Restriction 58
Side Effects of Diuretics 64
Practical Considerations for the
Use of Diuretics 70
Vasodilators
General Considerations of Vasodilators/
Nitrates/Hydralazine 74
Converting Enzyme Inhibitors 78
Digitalis
Digitalis: Indications and
Contraindications 88
Pharmacokinetics of Digitalis
Preparations/Clinical Use of Digitalis 90
Digitalis Toxicity 94

Experimental Pharmacologic Therapy
Beta Blockers ... 98
Experimental Inotropic Agents ... 100
Heart Failure in the ICU
General Considerations ... 102
Patterns of Hemodynamic Instability ... 106
Drug Treatment ... 110
Devices ... 122
Transplantation
Transplantation ... 126
Complications of Cardiac Transplantation ... 132
References
References ... 136

TABLES

TABLE 3.1 – Backward Failure/Congestive Symptoms/Left Ventricle ... 22
TABLE 3.2 – Backward Failure/Congestive Symptoms/Right Ventricle ... 23
TABLE 3.3 – Forward Flow/Low Output ... 23
TABLE 6.1 – Avid Sodium Retention in CHF ... 31
TABLE 6.2 – Mechanisms Contributing to Avid Sodium Retention ... 31
TABLE 7.1 – Mechanisms of Exercise Intolerance in CHF ... 33
TABLE 8.1 – Typical Precipitating Causes of CHF ... 38
TABLE 8.2 – New York Heart Association Classification of CHF ... 38
TABLE 9.1 – Causes of Heart Failure With a Normal Heart Size ... 43
TABLE 12.1 – Indications for Endomyocardial Biopsy ... 54
TABLE 12.2 – Difficulties With Myocardial Biopsy in Idiopathic Cardiomyopathy ... 54

TABLE 13.1 – Information Gained From Exercise Testing 57
TABLE 14.1 – Loop Diuretics 63
TABLE 14.2 – Non-Loop Diuretics 63
TABLE 14.3 – Potassium-Sparing Diuretics 63
TABLE 15.1 – Side Effects of Diuretics 66
TABLE 17.1 – Classification of Vasodilators 77
TABLE 18.1 – Pharmacokinetic Differences Between Captopril and Enalapril 87
TABLE 18.2 – Correlates of Increased Plasma Renin Activity 87
TABLE 20.1 – Pharmacokinetics of Digitalis Preparations 93
TABLE 21.1 – Extra Cardiac Manifestations of Digitalis Toxicity 97
TABLE 21.2 – Cardiac Manifestations of Digitalis Toxicity 97
TABLE 21.3 – Patients at Risk for Digitalis Toxicity 97
TABLE 25.1 – Patterns of Hemodynamic Instability 108
TABLE 26.1 – Nitroprusside 118
TABLE 26.2 – Nitroglycerin 118
TABLE 26.3 – Dopamine 118
TABLE 26.4 – Dobutamine 119
TABLE 26.5 – Amrinone (Inocor®) 119
TABLE 26.6 – Sympathomimetic Amines 120
TABLE 27.1 – Additional Measures in Refractory CHF 125
TABLE 27.2 – Intra-Aortic Balloon Pump 125
TABLE 28.1 – Indications for Cardiac Transplantation 131
TABLE 28.2 – Exclusion Criteria for Cardiac Transplantation 131
TABLE 29.1 – Complications of Cardiac Transplantation 133
TABLE 29.2 – University of Minnesota Cardiac Transplant Program 134

FIGURES

FIGURE 1.1 – Cardiac Dysfunction in Congestive Heart Failure 11
FIGURE 4.1 – Frank Starling Relationship – Dependence of Cardiac Function on Preload 26
FIGURE 4.2 – Relationship of Cardiac Output to Impedance 26
FIGURE 7.1 – Exercise Limitations of CHF 34
FIGURE 8.1 – Natural History of CHF 39

Center Index System

The purpose of the center index system is to enable readers to immediately locate all the information contained in the book. Tabs are provided with each center index so there is a direct connection between the center index and text. The text is organized in a sequential format to enable the reader to proceed to any area of the text without having to read through information not relevant to the situation.

#1 Definitions of Cardiac Failure

General Definitions

Cardiac failure is a clinical syndrome that is typically diagnosed when a patient presents with the symptoms of fatigue and dyspnea or breathlessness at rest or during exercise, accompanied by signs of cardiac impairment and/or fluid retention:

- Cardiac impairment:
  - Cardiomegaly
  - Ventricular diastolic gallop
  - Impaired contraction (echocardiogram nuclear heart scan, catheterization)
- Fluid retention:
  - Pulmonary venous congestion
  - Peripheral edema
  - Elevated jugular venous pressure

A simple definition of heart failure is that it is a syndrome characterized by:

- Impaired left ventricular function
- Reduced exercise tolerance
- High incidence of ventricular arrhythmias
- Shortened life expectancy

Previous definitions included the term "congestive" to describe the fluid retention that frequently accompanies heart failure. However, since many patients have heart failure in the absence of congestion, the preference is to delete the term "congestive" and use "heart failure" or "clinical heart failure."

All definitions of heart failure include a criterion of abnormal cardiac performance, or abnormal muscle function. There are two general types of abnormal muscle function:

- Systolic dysfunction
- Diastolic dysfunction

Performance of the left ventricle is defined by its ability to empty against a pressure load (systolic function) and its ability to fill at a low filling pressure (diastolic function). Systolic and diastolic function may be quantitated by both invasive and non-invasive techniques. It is also important to note that clinical heart failure (CHF) can be related to abnormalities in either systolic or diastolic dysfunction or a combination of both, as outlined in Figure 1.1.

Patients with CHF are described in Circle A of Figure 1.1. The most common cause of this clinical syndrome is systolic dysfunction, as represented by the overlap with Circle B (see Section #2).

The same clinical syndrome of CHF can be due to diastolic dysfunction, as represented by Circle C. Some patients with diastolic dysfunction have normal systolic function, e.g., hypertrophic cardiomyopathy. Other patients with CHF and diastolic dysfunction also have systolic dysfunction (shown as the overlap of all three circles), which is, in fact, the most common clinical combination.

It is possible for patients to have either systolic or diastolic dysfunction and not show signs or symptoms referable to the syndrome of CHF. This syndrome may be referred to as "asymptomatic left ventricular dysfunction" and is the subject of two multicenter trials currently in progress.

The distinctions noted above are important to consider when evaluating CHF patients (see Sections #12 through #18). Since the clinical syndrome of heart failure is due predominantly to left ventricular systolic dysfunction, however, the remainder of this book will concentrate on this population.

FIGURE 1.1 — **Cardiac Dysfunction in Congestive Heart Failure**

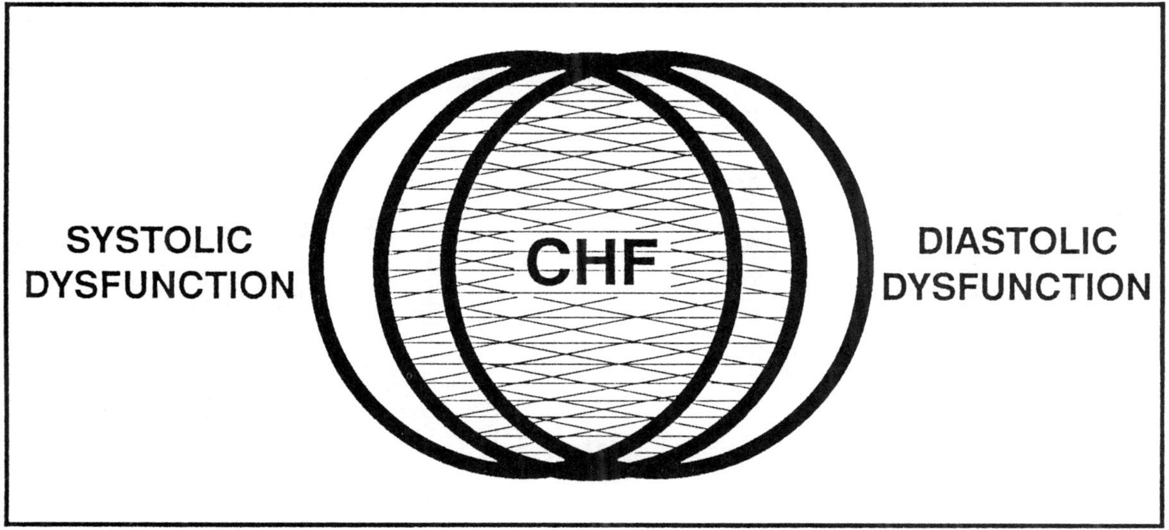

#2 Causes of Cardiac Failure and Cardiomyopathy

Although there are many potential causes of left ventricular systolic dysfunction that can result in cardiomyopathy and clinical symptoms of CHF, the most common are:

- Coronary artery disease
- Hypertension
- Valvular heart disease
- Infection
- Inflammation/collagen vascular disease
- Metabolic disease
- Toxic agents
- Infiltrative processes
- Fibroplastic processes
- Hematological diseases
- Genetic defects
- Postpartum cardiomyopathy
- Idiopathic cardiomyopathy

Coronary Artery Disease

Coronary artery disease is probably the most common cause of CHF in the United States, accounting for 40 to 50 percent of patients presenting with the clinical syndrome of heart failure. The typical patient with this "ischemic cardiomyopathy" might have a history of:

- Angina pectoris
- Previous myocardial infarction (MI)
- Coronary artery bypass surgery

In this case, the left ventricle is typically dilated, with marked increases in ventricular volumes and dimensions, and associated with an overall reduction in systolic function. The reduction in systolic function is usually due to regional rather than global wall motion abnormalities typical of the idiopathic cardiomyopathies. In selected cases, the reduction in left ventricular function is so severe that identification of regional abnormalities is difficult.

Special mention should be made of the important role of coronary angiography in making the diagnosis of "coronary artery disease and ischemic cardiomyopathy." Coronary angiography is required for the definitive diagnosis of "ischemic cardiomyopathy," though treatment decisions are not always affected by the results of the procedure. Some patients can have severe coronary artery disease without any antecedent documentation of angina or MI, and some patients develop severe left ventricular failure following a single transmural MI, likely influenced by peripheral vascular factors (see Sections #4 through #10).

In most cases, the treatment regimen of patients with a cardiomyopathy due to severe coronary artery disease will be the same as for patients with idiopathic cardiomyopathy and will include:

- Vasodilators
- Digitalis
- Diuretics

In selected cases, however, it is possible to demonstrate the presence of active myocardial ischemia, with or without a classic history of exertional angina, associated with reversible wall motion abnormalities during exercise gated blood pool scanning, or reversible perfusion defects on thallium scintigraphy (see Sections #9 through #13). Given suitable coronary anatomy, these patients may be treated with coronary artery bypass surgery or angioplasty, which can be associated with a marked reduction in their exercise limitation. Thus, coronary angiography may provide important information about the potential use of this treatment intervention.

Other clinical trials have confirmed that the survival of patients with severe three-vessel coronary disease and left ventricular dysfunction is considerably improved by bypass surgery when compared to medical therapy alone.

Hypertension

In the Framingham experience, hypertension is listed as one of the most common causes of the clinical syndrome of heart failure due to the deleterious effects of long-standing increases in impedance on left ventricular emptying and myocardial function. Diastolic dysfunction is also a common complication of hypertension.

A hypercontractile and hypertrophied ventricle in a hypertensive patient can also progress to a dilated, poorly-contractile ventricle. However, the exact mechanisms and time course of these pathophysiologic changes are not fully understood. Coronary artery disease frequently accompanies the hypertensive changes and may be an important component of the left ventricular dysfunction.

Valvular Heart Disease

Patients with volume overload due to long-standing aortic or mitral regurgitation may also develop severe left ventricular dilation and the clinical syndrome of CHF. Thus, CHF may be the end result of:

- Ischemic heart disease with papillary muscle dysfunction
- Rheumatic heart disease with aortic or mitral insufficiency
- Myxomatous mitral valve and mitral insufficiency

Aortic stenosis may also cause the clinical syndrome of heart failure, but, in most cases, the heart is not dilated until the final stages of the disease. Similarly, mitral stenosis can produce many features of heart failure though the heart size will be normal (see Section #3). These should not be confused with a dilated cardiomyopathy.

Infections

When the heart is involved in an inflammatory process caused by an infectious agent, a diagnosis of myocarditis can be made. Infectious agents may cause myocardial damage by:

- Direct invasion of the myocardium
- Production of a myocardial toxin
- An immunologic process

It is difficult to definitively diagnose an infectious cause of cardiomyopathy, however, given the limitations of currently available laboratory methods in identifying pathologic organisms and reproducing the clinical syndrome in laboratory animals. Cardiomyopathy has been associated with a number of bacterial pathogens, including:

- Diphtheria
- Salmonella
- Streptococcus (rheumatic fever)
- Meningococcus

Additionally, viral myocarditis may account for many cases of idiopathic cardiomyopathy. Several viral infections have been associated with myocarditis, including:

- Coxsackie A and B
- Echovirus
- Adenovirus
- Influenza
- Varicella

Other organisms have been associated with cardiac infections, though they are rare and atypical as causes of CHF. They include:

- Rickettsial infections
- Mycoplasma
- Tuberculosis
- Fungal infections

Chagas' disease, caused by *Trypanosoma cruzi*, is prevalent in Central and South America and is the most common cause of heart failure in the world.

Inflammatory Causes

The most important non-infectious collagen vascular disease resulting in myocardial damage is sarcoidosis. Heart involvement is a common accompaniment to the typical pulmonary and systemic manifestations of this disease, classically arrythmia and heart block, although heart failure has been described. Other collagen vascular diseases have been associated with cardiomyopathy, including systemic lupus erythematosus and polymyositis.

Inflammatory changes with lymphocytic myocardial infiltrates have been well described in many biopsy samples in patients with the recent onset of heart failure (see Section #12). Since the cause of these inflammatory changes is unknown, a diagnosis of "idiopathic inflammatory myocarditis" is commonly given.

Metabolic Causes

A dilated cardiomyopathy and CHF have been described in several metabolic disorders, including thiamine deficiency and kwashiorkor, as well as several endocrinologic problems, including:

- Acromegaly
- Thyrotoxicosis
- Myxedema
- Pheochromocytoma

Toxic Causes

A number of toxins have been associated with CHF, including cobalt poisoning and anthracycline chemotherapeutic agents, such as Adriamycin®. Since the recognition of these clinical syndromes, cobalt has been eliminated from beer processing and the dose of Adriamycin® has been reduced. Combined with prospective measurements of myocardial function, these entities are uncommon today.

One of the most interesting and common cardiomyopathies related to toxins is secondary to long-term consumption of alcohol. The exact mechanisms by which alcohol causes myocardial damage have not be elucidated but are generally associated with considerable quantities of alcohol ingested over an extended period.

Intriguing also is speculation about host modifications of responses to a specific toxin, since the more common response to excessive intake of alcohol is liver failure and not cardiac failure.

Infiltrative Causes

The most prominent of infiltrative disorders involving the heart are:

- Amyloidosis
- Hemochromatosis

Fibroplastic Causes

Fibroplastic causes include such entities as:

- Endomyocardial fibrosis
- Endocardial fibroelastosis

Hematologic Causes

Clinically apparent heart failure is uncommon with hematologic disorders, though cardiomyopathy has been associated with:

- Sickle cell anemia
- Polycythemia vera
- Thrombotic thrombocytopenic purpura

Genetic Causes

A familial cardiomyopathy with autosomal-dominant penetrance has been described, along with a high incidence of death due to severe arrhythmias and/or heart failure.

Postpartum Causes

Cardiomyopathy occurring in the last trimester of pregnancy or within six months after delivery is categorized as postpartum or peripartum cardiomyopathy.

Hypertrophic Cardiomyopathy

Hypertrophic cardiomyopathy is characterized by abnormal ventricular hypertrophy, arrhythmias, outflow obstruction (frequently), and restrictive physiology. On occasion, it may be associated with the clinical syndrome of heart failure, but systolic function is normally preserved.

Idiopathic Causes

A diagnosis of idiopathic dilated cardiomyopathy is made in the absence of an identifiable cause of ventricular dysfunction. Although it is a diagnosis of exclusion, it accounts for 40 to 50 percent of patients in most series of CHF.

#3 Clinical Signs and Symptoms

The clinical diagnosis of CHF is made by identification of the typical signs and symptoms. Two categories of pathophysiologic manifestations of heart failure, though somewhat arbitrary, must be considered:

- "Backward failure" – Symptoms are due to pulmonary and systemic congestion; these can be further divided into those primarily relating to:
  - Left ventricle
  - Right ventricle
- "Forward failure" – Symptoms are due to low cardiac output

Backward Failure

Left Ventricle

Backward failure of the left ventricle is primarily related to increased left ventricular end-diastolic pressure and increased pulmonary wedge pressure. Symptoms include:

- Dyspnea on exertion
- Paroxysmal nocturnal dyspnea
- Orthopnea
- Cough
- Wheezing
- Hemoptysis

Signs include:

- Cardiomegaly
- S3 gallop

- Rales
- Pleural effusions

Right Ventricle

Backward failure of the right ventricle is due to increased right ventricular end-diastolic pressure and increased right atrial pressure. Symptoms include:

- Right upper-quadrant discomfort (hepatic congestion)
- Abdominal distension and bloating
- Early satiety
- Ankle swelling

Signs include:

- Elevated jugular venous pressure
- Positive hepatojugular reflux
- Hepatomegaly
- Ascites
- Peripheral edema
- Splenomegaly (rare)

Forward Failure

Forward failure, or reduced forward flow, is due to low cardiac output. Symptoms include:

- Fatigue
- Weakness
- Lassitude
- Day and night reversal

Signs include:

- Weak pulses, decreased pulse pressure
- Peripheral vasoconstriction
- Cachexia and weight loss
- Cheyne-Stokes respirations
- Increased BUN/creatinine ratio

TABLE 3.1 – **Backward Failure/Congestive Symptoms/Left Ventricle**

Due to Increased Left Ventricular End-Diastolic Pressure and Increased Pulmonary Wedge Pressure
Symptoms: • Dyspnea on exertion • Paroxysmal nocturnal dyspnea • Orthopnea • Cough • Wheezing • Hemoptysis **Signs:** • Cardiomegaly • S3 Gallop • Rales • Pleural effusions

TABLE 3.2—**Backward Failure/Congestive Symptoms/Right Ventricle**

Due to Increased Right Ventricular End-Diastolic Pressure and Increased Right Atrial Pressure
Symptoms: • Right upper-quadrant discomfort (hepatic congestion) • Abdominal distension/bloating • Early satiety • Ankle swelling **Signs:** • Elevated jugular venous pressure • Positive hepatojugular reflux • Hepatomegaly • Ascites • Peripheral edema • Splenomegaly (rare)

TABLE 3.3—**Forward Flow/Low Output**

Symptoms:
- Fatigue
- Weakness
- Lassitude
- Day/night reversal

Signs:
- Weak pulses and decreased pulse pressure
- Peripheral vasoconstriction
- Cachexia/weight loss
- Cheyne Stokes respirations
- Increased BUN/creatinine ratio

#4 Starling Curve and Impedance/ Outflow Resistance

4.

The classic Frank Starling relationship (Figure 4.1) demonstrates the dependence of cardiac function upon preload. In normal individuals, the Starling relationship is steep, indicating that an increase in preload results in an increase in contractile force and cardiac output.

In contrast, the Starling curve of CHF patients is both flatter and more depressed. The typical CHF patient, Point A in Figure 4.1, has a marked increase in preload, manifested by an increased pulmonary wedge pressure and the usual symptoms of pulmonary congestion. Cardiac output often is decreased.

In general, cardiac function of the CHF patient is relatively independent of preload, a situation suggesting that maneuvers normally increasing preload do not lead to an increase in cardiac output because of the flat Starling curve. In fact, some maneuvers, such as volume loading, usually exacerbate the symptoms of pulmonary congestion.

Diuretics usually lead to a reduction in pulmonary wedge pressure and preload, though they do not increase cardiac output nor typically lessen the symptoms of low cardiac output (Figure 4.1, Arrow D). Vasodilators and inotropic agents, in contrast, can decrease preload and increase cardiac output (Figure 4.1, Arrows V and I, respectively), leading to an overall amelioration of the hemodynamic profile.

In contrast to the cardiac function-to-preload relationship is the cardiac output-to-impedance relationship. Impendance refers to the sum of the forces against which the ventricle must pump (see Figure 4.2). In normal subjects, the relationship of systemic outflow resistance and cardiac output is relatively flat, suggesting that interventions which normally increase or decrease outflow resistance do not affect cardiac output. Conversely, the curves in CHF patients are steep, indicating that, while the failing heart is preload-independent, it is sensitive to changes in afterload. Thus, interventions which reduce arteriolar tone and outflow resistance lead to increases in cardiac output. The steepness of the curve indicates that, for patients with the most severe forms of heart failure, the same reduction in resistance will lead to even greater increases in cardiac output.

FIGURES 4.1 and 4.2 ➡

FIGURE 4.1 – **Frank Starling Relationship – Dependence of Cardiac Function on Preload**

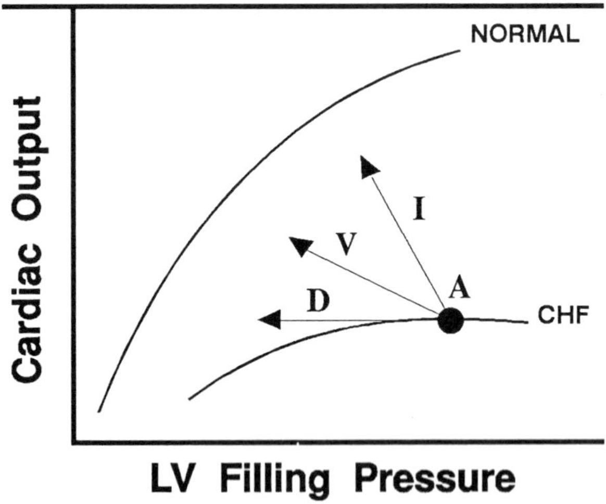

FIGURE 4.2 – **Relationship of Cardiac Output to Impedance**

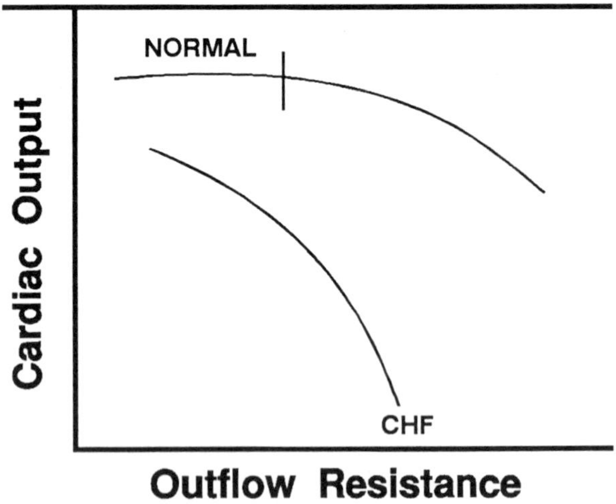

NOTES

#5 The Vicious Cycle of Heart Failure

CHF is usually initiated by a process that reduces left ventricular systolic function and cardiac output. To compensate for the reduction in cardiac output and to maintain constant mean arterial pressure, a reflex increase in systemic vascular resistance occurs.

Although the specific mechanisms by which
5. this vasoconstriction occurs are not known, activation of the following neurohormonal systems appears to be important:

- Renin-angiotensin system
- Sympathetic nervous system
- Arginine vasopressin pathway

Activation has been documented by several observations, including identification of elevated levels of plasma markers of these systems, including:

- Angiotensin II
- Norepinephrine
- Arginine vasopressin

Activation of these neurohormonal vasoconstrictor pathways can be viewed as beneficial during the initial stages of heart failure, since they help support blood pressure and the perfusion of vital organs. Over a period of time, however, these same beneficial pathways may:

- Lead to further reduction in renal blood flow
- Aggravate avid sodium-retention
- Increase systemic vascular resistance
- Impede left ventricular emptying

It is now well established that these developments have further adverse effects on left ventricular function, setting up a progressive, self-perpetuating, positive feedback cycle in which heart failure produces more heart failure and eventually results in an end-stage condition.

This is based on the finding that vasodilator therapy will dramatically improve the hemodynamic profile and survival rates of patients with heart failure by reversing the vasoconstriction caused by the neurohormonal systems.

Subsequent research has focused on interrupting this self-perpetuating, positive feedback cycle with vasodilators, as well as determining the optimal time to intervene.

#6 Salt and Water Reabsorption

6.

Avid sodium retention is one of the most important pathophysiologic mechanisms accounting for many symptoms of CHF patients (Table 6.1). Although a normal individual may consume up to six grams of sodium per day, he will eventually achieve neutral sodium balance, a state in which nearly all of the sodium taken into the body is excreted in the urine.

By contrast, avid sodium retention is a characteristic of CHF. In the CHF patient, the sodium excretion measured in the urine is significantly less than the amount of intake, possibly by one-third. This leaves the patient with a net positive sodium balance which, over an extended period, will lead to fluid accumulation and the typical signs and symptoms of CHF.

Many potential mechanisms contribute to the avid sodium retention state of CHF (Table 6.2), all of which appear to be important since blocking any one of these factors may improve sodium balance.

Treatments to minimize these signs and symptoms of heart failure (Table 6.1) include:

- Restricting sodium intake (see Sections #14 and #16)
- Using diuretics (see Sections #16 and #17)

These two treatment principles are interdependent. While diuretics may help a patient excrete excessive sodium, it is unlikely that his condition will significantly improve unless dietary sodium is restricted. Similarly, a patient who restricts his dietary intake of sodium can minimize symptoms with a smaller dose of diuretics.

TABLE 6.1 – **Avid Sodium Retention in CHF**

	Normal	*CHF*	*Treatment*
Sodium intake	6 gm	6 gm	Dietary sodium restriction
Sodium excretion	6 gm	4 gm	Diuretics
Sodium balance	0	+2 gm	

TABLE 6.2 – **Mechanisms Contributing to Avid Sodium Retention**

- Decreased cardiac output
- Decreased renal blood flow
- Activation of renin angiotensin system
- Increased aldosterone
- Increased vasopressin (ADH)
- Attenuated responses to atrial natriuretic factor

#7 Exercise Intolerance

A major pathophysiologic principle in CHF patients is exercise intolerance. CHF patients are not able to exercise normally (schematized in Figure 7.1) and are limited by symptoms of:

- Dyspnea on exertion
- Fatigue

7. During maximal exercise, normal subjects experience no major change in pulmonary wedge pressure while their cardiac output can increase four- to six-fold. At rest, CHF patients have a higher wedge pressure and lower cardiac output than normal subjects. During exercise, attenuated increases in cardiac output and exaggerated increases in pulmonary wedge pressure may occur, contributing to dyspnea and exertional fatigue.

This degree of exercise intolerance can be quantified using formal exercise testing (see Section #13). Weber et al have proposed a classification system based on functional aerobic capacity, as measured by oxygen consumption at peak exercise. In this classification, patients are identified as Class A if their oxygen consumption increases to greater than 20 ml/kg/minute at the end of exercise. Classes B through E represent gradually increasing functional limitations, with decreasing peak oxygen consumptions. The patients in Class E, those with the most severe forms of heart failure, have markedly limited exercise oxygen consumptions in the range of four to eight ml/kg/minute. It is important to note that normal subjects and CHF patients have an at-rest oxygen consumption of three to four ml/kg/minute. This means Class E patients are barely able to double their oxygen consumption during exercise.

The exact mechanisms which limit exercise performance in CHF patients are currently under intense investigation. Table 7.1 lists the two categories of mechanisms suggested as causes.

TABLE 7.1 – **Mechanisms of Exercise Intolerance in CHF**

Cardiac Causes

- Inability to appropriately increase heart rate
- Insufficient cardiac reserve
- Increased afterload
- Myocardial ischemia

Peripheral Vascular Factors

- Inability to appropriately vasodilate and increase blood flow to skeletal muscle
- Shunting of blood
- Possible peripheral nutritive defect
- Abnormal autonomic reflexes

FIGURE 7.1 – **Exercise Limitations of CHF**

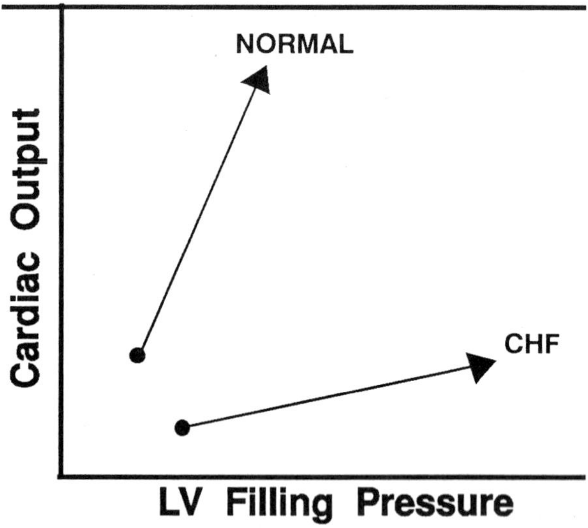

NOTES

#8 Precipitating Causes of CHF/Survival

Precipitating Causes

When a patient presents with decompensated heart failure, any potential precipitating cause(s) must be determined. (See Table 8.1 for a list of typical precipitating causes.) By the process of eliminating precipitating causes, clinical stability can be obtained more readily.

The evaluation should include:

- Patient history
- Physical examination
- Laboratory testing

Survival

8.

Figure 8.1 schematizes the natural history of patients with left ventricular dysfunction and CHF, relating the percent of patient survival to the time of onset of myocardial disease.

As the disease progresses and the patient moves from New York Heart Class I to Class IV heart failure (Table 8.2), symptoms of CHF develop initially during stress and subsequently at rest. With the development of symptoms, survival rates decrease.

Causes of death include:

- Ventricular arrhythmias
- Progressive end-stage pump failure

The decrease in survival rates can be dramatic, as indicated by the steep curve in Figure 8.1. Studies have repeatedly demonstrated that

New York Heart Class III to IV heart failure patients referred to tertiary care centers have high mortality rates, with an estimated two-year survival rate of approximately 30 to 40 percent. This high mortality rate, greater than that of many cancer patients, highlights the lethal nature of CHF.

Many investigators have attempted to describe the most important prognostic factors affecting the survival of CHF patients. The disparate results are difficult to compare, given the differences in patient populations and other measurement techniques. As anticipated, generally the more severe the left ventricular dysfunction or symptoms of heart failure, the worse the prognosis. Several interventions have been shown to favorably affect the survival curve of CHF patients, including:

- Cardiac transplantation (see Sections #28 and #29)
- Vasodilators (see Sections #17 through #20)

Tables 8.1 and 8.2
Figure 8.1 →

TABLE 8.1 – **Typical Precipitating Causes of CHF**

1. Dietary noncompliance
2. Medication noncompliance
3. Infection
4. Arrhythmia
5. Thromboembolic complication
6. Myocardial infarction or ischemia
7. Anemia
8. Hypothyroidism and hyperthyroidism
9. Pregnancy

TABLE 8.2 – **New York Heart Association Classification**

Class I	No undue symptoms on ordinary activity No limitation of physical activity
Class II	Slight limitation of physical activity Patient comfortable at rest
Class III	Marked limitation of physical activity Patient comfortable at rest
Class IV	Discomfort with any physical activity Symptoms of cardiac insufficiency at rest

FIGURE 8.1 – **Natural History of CHF**

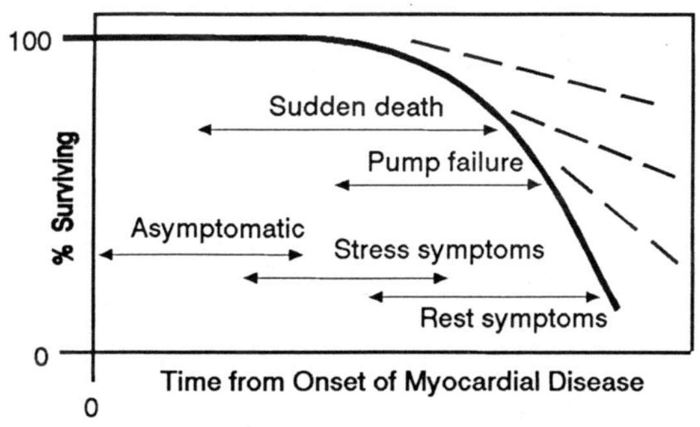

#9 Laboratory Assessment I: Electrocardiogram/Chest X-Ray

Laboratory Assessment

The laboratory workup of the CHF patient will usually include an electrocardiogram and chest x-ray (see below), but most patients will also have either an echocardiogram and/or a nuclear heart scan to quantify left ventricular dysfunction (see Section #10). More invasive and sophisticated tests will depend on the uncertainty of diagnosis after these routine tests or on the need to evaluate the effectiveness of therapy.

Electrocardiogram

Electrocardiography should be performed in all patients presenting with the clinical syndrome of CHF. This excellent screening technique has the advantages of:

- Being safe
- Being inexpensive
- Showing signs of previous myocardial infarction
- Possibly detecting arrhythmias

The disadvantages are that it:

- Is non-specific
- Offers no quantification of ventricular function

The electrocardiogram provides information on a large number of abnormalities, including:

- Evidence of left ventricular hypertrophy
- Q waves, indicating previous myocardial infarction
- Conduction delays and/or bundle branch blocks
- Left or right atrial abnormalities
- Left axis deviation

These findings lack specificity, however, since most patients with cardiomyopathy and heart failure have several of these abnormalities. Because the electrocardiogram provides no quantification of ventricular function, other imaging tests are required.

Arrhythmias should be noted, since they frequently:

- Lead to exacerbations of heart failure, e.g., recent onset of atrial fibrillation (see Section #8)
- May indicate digitalis toxicity, e.g., paroxysmal atrial tachycardia (see Section #21)

If intermittent arrhythmias are suspected, the electrocardiogram can be supplemented with 24-hour ambulatory monitoring. Recent experience has also suggested that such monitoring can:

- Identify patients with frequent and complex ventricular ectopy who are at high risk for:
  - Sustained ventricular tachyarrhythmias
  - Sudden cardiac death
- Help to determine if antiarrhythmic drug therapy or referral for electrophysiologic testing is necessary

Chest X-Ray

The chest x-ray is another simple laboratory test which should be performed as a screening test for all patients with heart failure. The chest x-ray offers the advantages of:

- Safety
- Providing information on pulmonary venous congestion
- Demonstrating cardiomegaly

Disadvantages are that the chest x-ray:

- Is non-specific
- Offers no quantification of left ventricular systolic function
- Correlates poorly with left ventricular size

The chest x-ray may help quantify congestive signs and symptoms by the presence of:

- Pulmonary venous congestion
- Kerly B lines
- Pulmonary vascular redistribution
- Pleural effusions

Most importantly, the chest x-ray provides the first clue for the diagnosis of chronic left ventricular systolic dysfunction by indicating the presence or absence of cardiomegaly (see Section #2). A patient with the clinical syndrome of heart failure but a normal heart size, therefore, might prompt an investigation of other disorders (Table 9.1).

NOTES

#11 Laboratory Assessment III: Cardiac Catheterization

In most cases, the diagnosis of heart failure can be confirmed by the tests mentioned in Sections #9 and #10. However, in some cases with concomitant pulmonary disease or in patients in whom it is not possible to obtain satisfactory images of the heart, cardiac catheterization may be necessary.

Right Heart Catheterization

Right heart catheterization aids in diagnosis of heart failure by the accurate documentation of:

- Reduced cardiac output
- Increased pulmonary artery pressure
- Increased pulmonary wedge pressure

These parameters can only be estimated by echocardiography. Furthermore, in selected patients, monitoring cardiac output and cardiac pressures during exercise may help to determine the cause of exercise-induced dyspnea.

Finally, right heart catheterization may help assess the adequacy and efficacy of diuretic, vasodilator, and inotropic drug therapy in terms of preload and cardiac output with a precision and sensitivity that are not possible with non-invasive methods.

Right heart catheterization has the disadvantages of being:

- Invasive
- Associated with a number of complications, including:

- Arrhythmias
- Thrombosis
- Infection

- Difficult to perform serially
- Expensive

Left Heart Catheterization

Left heart catheterization is considered the "gold standard" for:

- The measurement of left ventricular systolic function
- Determining the presence and severity of mitral regurgitation

Coronary angiography is the definitive test for determining the presence of obstructive coronary disease. This is important in assessing the role of coronary disease in the pathogenesis of the underlying cardiac dysfunction, since coronary artery bypass surgery is frequently helpful in patients with suitable coronary anatomy who have signs or symptoms of recurrent bouts of ischemia. Several studies have shown that bypass surgery in these patients, especially with moderate to severe reductions in ejection fraction, can be performed with an acceptable perioperative mortality and is associated with improved long-term survival rates, compared to medical treatment alone.

Based on this experience, greater numbers of patients undergo coronary angiography; in the past, the procedure had little impact on therapeutic interventions because surgery was typically not considered if the ejection fraction was less than 35 percent.

This procedure is helpful even when bypass surgery is not recommended for a patient. It offers information on coronary obstructive lesions, aiding in treatment design strategies for patients with severe exercise-induced dyspnea and in whom both ischemia and increased wall stress may be important. These patients frequently benefit from the addition of nitrate therapy and occasionally benefit from calcium channel blockers.

Disadvantages of the procedure are that it:

- Is invasive
- Involves a number of risks
- Is expensive

NOTES

#12 Laboratory Assessment IV: Endomyocardial Biopsy

Endomyocardial biopsy is frequently used in the evaluation of CHF patients (Table 12.1). Its most prominent clinical use, however, is in the monitoring of cardiac transplant rejection, since there may be significant pathologic evidence of rejection prior to any clinical manifestations. Therefore, routine biopsies are repeated at frequent intervals for all transplant patients.

The biopsy is also useful in cases of suspected myocarditis, in which the demonstration of a cellular infiltrate, due to an infectious or non-infectious inflammatory process, is the typical finding that may prompt consideration of the use of immunosuppressant drugs.

Finally, several secondary cardiomyopathies, e.g., amyloid, can be definitively diagnosed by endomyocardial biopsy.

Endomyocardial biopsy has undergone several improvements recently and can now be performed as an outpatient procedure with a low incidence of complications, e.g., perforation, arrhythmias. The most important factor in this procedure, however, is not the skill of the catheterization personnel but the experience of the surgical pathology department to recognize pertinent abnormalities.

However, there are several reasons why endomyocardial biopsy is not routinely performed in the work-up of all patients with a suspected cardiomyopathy (Table 12.2). First, there is a disappointingly low sensitivity of positive results in patients with heart failure. This may be related to the fact that specimens are only one to two mm in thickness and can only be obtained from the endocardium; inflammatory changes can be patchy and involve small percentages of the total myocardium. Due to this sampling problem, the yield of diagnosis is small:

- Less than 30 percent in myocarditis
- Less than 15 percent in patients with chronic dilated cardiomyopathy

Another drawback is that the majority of the pathologic findings are non-specific, including:

- Myocyte hypertrophy
- Nuclear enlargement
- Hyperchromaticity
- Interstitial fibrosis

Additionally, there is great interobserver variability, as demonstrated in a recent study by Shanes et al. In this study, representative slides were independently reviewed by several different cardiac pathologists. There was little concordance of test results.

Based on these conclusions, endomyocardial biopsy is recommended in the workup of CHF patients when the onset of symptoms is less than six months prior to the time of evaluation. If the duration of symptoms is greater than six months, the chance of finding a cellular infiltrate that would prompt a treatment intervention is small. The presence of a cellular infiltrate raises a therapeutic dilemma. Although steroids and immunosuppresants have been used in such instances, there is as yet no data indicating that such therapy improves cardiac function long-term or overall prognosis.

TABLE 12.1 – **Indications for Endomyocardial Biopsy**

- Suspected cardiac allograft rejection
- Suspected myocarditis
- Detection and monitoring of doxorubicin cardiotoxicity
- Diagnosis of secondary cardiomyopathies

TABLE 12.2 – **Difficulties with Myocardial Biopsy in Idiopathic Cardiomyopathy**

1. Low sensitivity

   A. 1 to 2 mm specimens – Endocardial-only sampling
   B. Patchy process that may involve only 5% of myocardium
   C. Yield in myocarditis: Less than 30%
   D. Yield in idiopathic dilated cardiomyopathy: Less than 15%

2. Findings are nonspecific including myocyte hypertrophy and disarray, nuclear enlargement, and hyperchromaticity and interstitial fibrosis

3. Interobserver variability

NOTES

#13 Laboratory Assessment V: Exercise Testing

Exercise testing is probably underutilized in the evaluation of patients with heart failure, likely because of the perception that it may be too difficult for the elderly or brittle patient to perform. However, several less intensive exercise protocols can be employed so that even a maximal exercise test can be safely tolerated by most patients.

The information gained from an exercise test is listed in Table 13.1. Standard measurements include those of:

- Blood pressure
- Heart rate
- Electrocardiogram
- Exercise duration

By making these measurements, the adequacy of cardiac reserve and the overall functional status of the patient can be quantified and potential myocardial ischemia can be identified. The extent of cardiac functional limitation can only be assessed during exercise, as there is frequently a disparity from a patient's descriptions of his limitations. These tests are reliable and reproducible and can be followed serially to assess the efficacy of therapeutic interventions.

13. Many researchers have used analysis of expired air for the measurement of oxygen consumption and carbon dioxide production. These data give additional information on peak oxygen consumption and anaerobic threshold, which may be more objective and sensitive parameters of a patient's

cardiac reserve. Since these tests require the use of sensitive equipment operated by experienced personnel, they are generally confined to sophisticated exercise laboratories.

TABLE 13.1 – **Information Gained from Exercise Testing**

- Quantification of cardiac reserve during exercise
- Quantification of functional status
- Quantification of volitional effort

#14 Dietary Sodium Restriction

There is no doubt that diuretics offer effective treatment of CHF patients. Diuretics:

- Inhibit the ability of the kidney to reabsorb sodium and chloride
- Increase sodium and water excretion from the body
- Reduce fluid accumulation
- Reduce symptoms related to excessive vascular fluid

Although diuretics are important therapy for many CHF patients, these drugs should always be combined with dietary sodium restriction (see Section #6), since diuretics will not satisfactorily control edema formation without such intake restriction. Generally, dietary sodium intake should be restricted to 2,000 to 3,000 mg per day, depending on the severity of edema formation. Patients should be counseled to:

- Recognize that most foods contain salt
- Remove the salt shaker from the house
- Avoid high-salt foods and condiments
- Substitute natural herbs and spices for salt
- Keep a daily log of sodium intake

Sodium intake cannot be eliminated completely, since most foods contain sodium naturally. Thus, the patient's goal should be to restrict rather than eliminate sodium. It is recommended

that the salt shaker be removed from the dining table and kitchen, because one teaspoon of salt contains up to 2,300 mg of sodium, the total daily allowance. Large quantities of sodium are consumed in even small "pinches" of salt, causing and/or promoting edema formation.

Patients often claim that they do not add salt to their diets but that they still have "refractory" edema formation. It is likely that their diets include high-salt foods. High-salt foods that need to be avoided or substantially limited in such patients' diets include:

- Processed luncheon meats
- Frankfurters, sausages
- Condiments
- Snacks
- Canned vegetables
- Restaurant foods

Processed luncheon meats, frankfurters, sausages, and condiments use concentrated quantities of salt as a preservative and seasoning. Canned vegetables also contain substantial amounts of salt, while frozen or fresh vegetables contain only minimal amounts.

It is particularly important for patients who have been stabilized on diuretic therapy not to indulge in "binge" salt eating, since this may result in acute circulatory congestion whose adverse effects may persist far longer than the fluid overload.

Dining in restaurants may be particularly difficult for the CHF patient, since salt is liberally used in restaurant food to heighten taste. Despite the increase in the health consciousness of diners and restaurant owners, it is often difficult to maintain a sodium-restricted diet when dining out. One Big Mac, for example, contains more than 1,200 mg of sodium. If a patient must eat out frequently, he should be encouraged to select fresh foods, items without sauces, broiled meats, and salads with oil and vinegar rather than cream dressings. The flavor of foods may be enhanced by the use of natural herbs and spices and salt substitutes.

It is advisable for patients to keep daily, accurate logs of their sodium intake. Many paperback books list sodium contents of foods (including brand name items) to aid accurate record keeping. This gives the patient control and flexibility over his meal planning.

The caveat with dietary sodium restriction is that food should always be palatable, since eating pleasures are a vital part of the "quality of life."

It is equally important that patients take in the calories, proteins, and vitamins necessary for overall nutrition maintenance and for the avoidance of "cardiac cachexia," which frequently accompanies end-stage heart failure.

Loop Diuretics

Loop diuretics are potent drugs that work by inhibiting chloride transport in the thick, ascending loop of Henle, leading to marked increases in sodium excretion. Given the typical severity of the sodium retention in heart failure and reductions in renal blood flow and glomerular filtration rates, potent loop diuretics are commonly prescribed to initiate and maintain an adequate diuresis. Loop diuretics commonly used are listed in Table 14.1.

All loop diuretics are reasonably well absorbed from the gastrointestinal tract, although bioavailability and absorption rates are highly variable. It is frequently advisable to give first doses of loop diuretics intravenously to patients with severe gastrointestinal edema to ensure 100 percent bioavailability; oral preparations may be used once bowel edema has been satisfactorily decreased and gastrointestinal absorption is consistent.

All loop diuretics are roughly equivalent in terms of efficacy and toxicity, though ototoxicity may be more common with ethacrynic acid. The choice of loop diuretic type is frequently based on the physician's personal preference and his experience with the drug.

Non-Loop Diuretics

These agents (Table 14.2) act by inhibiting sodium reabsorption in the early part of the distal convoluted tubule but, when given alone, are typically less potent than loop diuretics and less effective as single-drug therapy in the control of edema and fluid accumulation in CHF patients. These drugs also tend to be significantly less effective in patients with severe renal insufficiency or when the glomerular filtration rate is less than 30 ml per minute.

However, non-loop diuretics are potent adjuncts to loop diuretics and will synergistically augment their diuretic action. Typically, in a patient requiring greater than 120 mg of Lasix®, 50 mg of hydrochlorathiazide or 5 mg of metolazone may initiate a satisfactory diuresis.

Potassium-Sparing Diuretics

Potassium-sparing diuretics are relatively less potent than loop and proximal tubule agents and therefore are not commonly used in patients with refractory CHF. However, since these patients are typically on high doses of loop diuretics and find it difficult to tolerate large doses of potassium supplements, potassium-sparing diuretics may help reduce potassium losses, increasing total body potassium and reducing the need for potassium supplements.

Spironolactone is a specific antagonist of aldosterone, which is frequently elevated in CHF patients due to activation of the renin-angiotensin system. The diuretic and potassium-sparing effects are not immediate; prolonged administration (several weeks) may be necessary to achieve full therapeutic effect.

Triamterene and amiloride inhibit sodium reabsorption by the distal tubule and collecting duct, and efficacy is independent of the presence of aldosterone. These relatively weak diuretics are occasionally helpful in reducing potassium wastage.

All potassium-sparing diuretics can be associated with hyperkalemia, especially in those patients receiving converting enzyme inhibitors. For this reason, potassium levels should be closely monitored.

TABLE 14.1 – **Loop Diuretics**

Name	Brand Name	Usual Dosage	Duration of Action
Furosemide	Lasix	20 to 240 mg/day	4 to 6 hours
Ethacrynic acid	Edecrin	50 to 200 mg/day	6 to 8 hours
Bumetanide	Bumex	1 to 10 mg/day	6 to 18 hours

TABLE 14.2 – **Non-Loop Diuretics**

Name	Brand Name	Usual Dosage
Hydrochlorothiazide	HydroDIURIL	25 to 100 mg/day
Chlorthalidone	Hygroton	25 to 100 mg/day
Metolazone	Zaroxolyn Diulo	2.5 to 10 mg

TABLE 14.3 – **Potassium-Sparing Diuretics***

Name	Brand Name	Dose
Spironolactone	Aldactone	25 to 200 mg/day
Triamterene	Dyrenium	37.5 to 200 mg/day
Amiloride	Midamor	2.5 to 10 mg/day

*Usually used in combination with a loop or non-loop diuretic

#15 Side Effects of Diuretics

Excessive diuresis may reduce effective arterial blood volume, which may further reduce renal blood flow and exacerbate renal insufficiency. It should be emphasized that volume contraction is not an adverse effect of diuresis per se but does represent an effect based on pharmacologic activity. Clinically, this may be apparent by:

- A decrease in blood pressure
- An increase in BUN/creatinine ratio
- Metabolic alkalosis
- A decrease in daily urine output
- Decreased skin turgor
- Decreased moisture of mucus membranes

Typical symptoms include:

- Fatigue
- Weakness
- Orthostatic light-headedness

This complication usually responds to the temporary discontinuation of diuretics but may require sodium and volume repletion either orally or intravenously, depending on the severity of the volume contraction.

Vasodilators may also exacerbate the adverse effects associated with volume contraction. Therefore, any decreases in blood pressure or orthostatic symptoms due to the diuretic-induced volume depletion may be intensified in patients taking vasodilators (see Sections #17 through #20).

Other complications associated with diuretics have been well recognized in patients under long-term diuretic treatment for hypertension. These complications, which should be closely monitored, include:

- Gout
- Diabetes
- Metabolic alkalosis
- Hearing loss
- Changes in lipid metabolism

Also important is the fact that diuretics can activate the renin-angiotensin system, even without marked volume depletion and even in patients with mild heart failure, thereby increasing:

- Angiotensin II mediated vasoconstriction
- Aldosterone

These conditions potentially exacerbate the clinical syndrome of CHF.

A classic study by Ikram et al demonstrated that continued use of diuretics, though initially helpful in decompensated heart failure, was associated with further decreases in cardiac output, likely secondary to increased vasoconstriction. It has been speculated that chronic administration of diuretics is an important contributor to the progressive self-perpetuating cycle of heart failure. Therefore, it is advisable that physicians prescribe only the smallest doses of diuretics necessary for the control of edema and normalities of central venous pressure.

TABLE 15.1 – **Side Effects of Diuretics**

1. Volume contraction
2. Renal insufficiency
3. Gout
4. Diabetes
5. Hearing loss
6. Metabolic alkalosis
7. Hyperlipidemia
8. Activation of the renin-angiotensin system

NOTES

CENTER

No.	Topic	Section
1.	Definitions	General Information
2.	Causes of Cardiac Failure and Cardiomyopathy	
3.	Clinical Signs and Symptoms	Signs and Symptoms
4.	Starling Curve and Impedance/ Outflow Resistance	Patho-Physiology
5.	Vicious Cycle of Heart Failure	
6.	Salt and Water Reabsorption	
7.	Exercise Intolerance	
8.	Precipitating Causes/Survival	
9.	Electrocardiogram/Chest X-Ray	Laboratory Assessment
10.	Echocardiogram/Nuclear Heart Scan	
11.	Cardiac Catheterization	
12.	Endomyocardial Biopsy	
13.	Exercise Testing	
14.	Dietary Sodium Restriction	Diuretics
15.	Side Effects	

INDEX

Section	Topic	Tab
Diuretics	Practical Considerations	16.
Vasodilators	General Considerations/ Nitrates/Hydralazine	17.
	Converting Enzyme Inhibitors	18.
Digitalis	Indications/Contraindications	19.
	Pharmacokinetics of Digitalis Preparations/Clinical Uses	20.
	Digitalis Toxicity	21.
Experimental Pharmacologic Therapy	Beta Blockers	22.
	Experimental Inotropic Agents	23.
Heart Failure in the ICU	General Considerations	24.
	Patterns of Hemodynamic Instability	25.
	Drug Treatment	26.
	Devices	27.
Trans-plantation	General Information/Indications/ Exclusions	28.
	Complications	29.
References	References	30.

#16 Practical Considerations for the Use of Diuretics

The patient requiring diuretic therapy will experience many of the typical signs and symptoms of heart failure. These may include:

- Dyspnea on exertion
- Abdominal distension
- Increased jugular venous pulse with positive hepatojugular reflux
- Rales/pleural effusions
- Peripheral edema

For these patients, dietary sodium restriction should be maintained. Furosemide may be begun at 40 mg per day and, if fluid accumulation is severe, increased to 120 to 240 mg per day, with the effective dose monitored by:

- Daily weight—As edema fluid decreases, the patient's weight should decrease
- Physical examination
- Laboratory tests of:
  - Serum creatinine and BUN
  - Electrolytes
  - Uric acid
  - Glucose

If patients demonstrate signs of volume contraction, usually manifested by increases in the BUN/creatinine ratio, the diuretic dosage should be decreased.

If high doses of furosemide are unsuccessful in reducing fluid, progressive steps may be taken to treat the edema. The patient should be:

- Reviewed for dietary sodium intake
- Given a non-loop diuretic, such as hydrochlorothiazide or metolazone
- Given intravenous diuretics, if poor absorption of orally-administered diuretics is suspected (due to gastrointestinal edema)
- Given low doses of dopamine (see Section #26) to selectively increase renal plasma flow

Once "dry" weight and an acceptable reduction in peripheral edema are achieved, the dosage of diuretics should be reduced. Dietary sodium restriction should be maintained, and diuretics should be increased only when necessary to control the edema. The "end point" of diuretic therapy may also be assessed by normalizing the cardiac filling pressure, as manifested by the jugular venous pulse, a method which has the added advantage of optimizing the overall hemodynamics of the CHF patient.

The long-term management of patients who typically experience episodic fluid accumulation, likely secondary to dietary indiscretion associated with binge salt intake, presents another difficult problem. It is useful to keep the dose of the loop diuretic constant and to add a non-loop diuretic on a PRN basis for one to three days, depending on the severity of sodium accumulation, thereby avoiding the need to continually adjust the dose of loop diuretic. This combination, however, is synergistic in potassium wastage, meaning that a potassium supplement must also be increased in this therapy regimen.

Use of Diuretics as Single-Drug Therapy

Diuretics have been used as single-drug therapy for the relief of many disabling symptoms typical of CHF because of their time-tested effectiveness. Recent evidence from large clinical trials, however, suggests that diuretics may not be beneficial as single-drug therapy.

Patients receiving vasodilating therapy, in addition to diuretics, have shown important increases in exercise performance and New York Association classification, as well as fewer hospitalizations and emergency room visits, as compared to patients receiving diuretics alone.

Furthermore, the V-HeFT and CONSENSUS trials have conclusively shown that vasodilators can prolong survival in diuretic-treated patients. The mechanism of this additional benefit over that of diuretics alone has not been fully defined, though it may relate to excessive vasoconstriction and adverse activation of the renin angiotensin.

Because of these findings, diuretic therapy is rarely used as single-drug therapy and is often combined with vasodilators and digoxin in the initial treatment of CHF patients.

NOTES

#17 General Considerations of Vasodilators/Nitrates/Hydralazine

Vasodilators

There are a number of vasodilators available for use by CHF patients. One simple classification is based on the dominant site of action, including venodilation and arterial dilation (Table 17.1).

The venodilators increase the capacitance of the veins and redistribute blood away from the central circulation. The decrease in ventricular filling and preload is effective in relieving systemic and pulmonary venous congestion.

In contrast, the arterial dilators decrease vascular resistance and impedance to left ventricular ejection, thereby leading to an increase in stroke volume and cardiac output. Typically, however, pure arterial dilators have little effect on preload.

The combined dilators have dual actions on the venous and arterial systems.

Though many vasodilators are available, only three have been shown to be clinically useful in the long-term treatment of patients with chronic CHF. These are:

- Nitrates
- Hydralazine
- Converting enzyme inhibitors

Nitrates

Nitrates are predominantly venodilators, which lead to decreases in preload, as manifested by decreases in right atrial pressure and pulmonary wedge pressure. At high doses, nitrates can have arteriolar dilating action, leading to minor decreases in blood pressure and systemic vascular resistance associated with an increase in cardiac output.

These drugs can be administered in many different forms:

- The sublingual or buccal forms, which have a duration of action of less than two hours
- The oral form, including isosorbide dinitrate, which is well absorbed but undergoes a first-pass effect by the liver. A typical dose is 10 to 40 mg with a duration of action of four to six hours
- Nitroglycerin, administered topically in the form of an ointment or a sustained-release patch

Nitrates improve exercise tolerance in CHF patients and may also improve coronary perfusion in patients with co-existent angina. However, since nitrates only modestly increase cardiac output in heart failure, they are often combined with an arterial dilator, such as hydralazine, for chronic management.

Recent interest in the problem of hemodynamic attenuation of the response to nitrates has led to concern about long-term benefits of chronic therapy. The mechanism of such tachyphylaxis may be related to a loss of sulfhydryl groups required for the generation of nitric oxide, which is an endothelial derived relaxing factor (EDRF).

Nitrates should be administered on a schedule that provides an eight- to 10-hour daily interval without drugs. With oral isosorbide dinitrate, this can be accomplished with an evening dose no later than 10:00 p.m. and a morning dose at 8:00 a.m. When transdermal preparations are used, the drug probably should be removed for at least six to eight hours at night to maintain full responsiveness.

Generally, nitrates are well tolerated, with the most common side effect being headaches, which frequently attenuate over time. Hypotension occurs, as with any other vasodilator, especially in people with low-filling pressures who cannot tolerate venous return reductions.

Hydralazine

Hydralazine is a direct-acting vasodilator with mainly arterial action producing large increases in cardiac output. Since the drug does not affect preload, it is usually combined with nitrates in order to achieve a balanced effect.

The hemodynamic effect of hydralazine is dose-related, with higher doses generally leading to incremental effects. Therefore, it is difficult to define an "optimal" dose in some patients. A daily regimen of 200 to 300 mg in two to four divided doses usually produces a favorable hemodynamic effect without undue side effects.

Hydralazine is metabolized by acetylation and is, therefore, affected by acetylator phenotype. Drug-induced lupus syndrome may occur in slow acetylators, but the incidence is less than one percent in CHF patients using this treatment regimen.

In addition to their effects on the signs and symptoms of heart failure, the combination of hydralazine and isosorbide dinitrate has been shown in the V-HeFT trial to prolong survival (see Section #16).

Other Vasodilators

Other clinically available vasodilators have been shown to have a favorable hemodynamic effect in heart failure but have not been shown to exert a long-term beneficial clinical response. Prazosin, an alpha-1 antagonist, exerts an arterial and venous dilating effect but did not have a long-term beneficial effect in the V-HeFT trial.

Minoxidil is a potent arterial vasodilator that markedly augments cardiac output. Its chronic use may be associated with sodium retention. Long-term benefits of this drug have not been demonstrated.

The calcium antagonists, particularly the dihydropyridine drugs (nifedipine, nicardipine) exert potent vasodilator effects. However, they may also have a negative inotropic effect in patients with heart failure, and adequate studies of efficacy in heart failure have not been conducted.

TABLE 17.1 – **Classification of Vasodilators**

Venodilators	Dilators Arterial	Combined Dilators
Nitrates	Hydralazine Nifedipine Minoxidil	Converting Enzyme Inhibitors Prazosin Nitroprusside

#18 Converting Enzyme Inhibitors

Converting enzyme inhibitors (CEIs) now are widely used as the vasodilator of choice for CHF patients. A number of studies have been conducted which demonstrate the clinical efficacy and safety of this drug.

Acute Hemodynamic Effects

CEIs produce a consistent decrease in systemic vascular resistance, with a maximal reduction ranging from 10 to 20 percent due to a reduction in angiotensin II-mediated vasoconstriction. This is associated with reduction of a mean arterial pressure ranging from seven to 25 percent that is generally well-tolerated, even when starting with a relatively low blood pressure.

The reduction in impedance results in:

- Improvement of cardiac output
- Improvement in stroke volume, with increases between 15 to 40 percent at peak effect
- Significant reductions (15 to 40 percent) in:
  - Pulmonary artery pressure
  - Pulmonary capillary wedge pressure
  - Right atrial pressure

The effects on heart rate after the administration of a CEI have been variable, with most studies showing either no change or slight reductions in heart rate; this effect, however, is difficult to interpret because of baseline abnormalities in the autonomic nervous system control of heart rate in CHF patients.

Generally, the magnitude of the hemodynamic responses after the first-dose administration of either captopril or enalapril appears to be closely related to the baseline level of renin-angiotensin system activity. Thus, there are significant correlations between baseline plasma renin activity and the magnitude of the changes in:

- Systemic vascular resistance
- Pulmonary wedge pressure
- Cardiac index

This information can be helpful when anticipating acute reductions in blood pressure, i.e., if one is able to estimate plasma renin activity, one may predict which patients might have large reductions in blood pressure following the first dose of CEI. A low serum sodium (<130 mEq/L) serves as a useful marker for a high plasma renin activity.

Hormonal Effects of ACE Inhibitors

Since angiotensin II has negative feedback inhibition on renin secretion, a consistent effect of all ACE inhibitors is an increase in plasma renin activity. Also, since angiotensin II is a potent stimulus for aldosterone secretion from the adrenal gland, the reduction in angiotensin II results in a reduction in plasma aldosterone levels. Consequently, natriuresis and potassium retention may be additional important benefits for CHF patients. The effects of ACE inhibitors on levels of circulating norepinephrine are variable. Some studies have demonstrated that circulating plasma norepiniphrine in CHF patients treated with CEI is decreased, possibly secondary to overall hemodynamic improvement or to the reduction in angiotensin II-stimulated norepinephrine secretion. It is currently undetermined whether this will have important implications for the long-term survival of CHF patients.

Clinical Effects of CEI

At least two-thirds of patients treated with CEI report improvement in symptoms as assessed by subjective reporting and the New York Heart Association functional classification. This improvement in functional classification can be confirmed by formal exercise testing, as measured by total exercise duration during treadmill or bicycle ergometer testing. Improvements in functional capacity and exercise capability have been reported in long-term, randomized, double-blind, placebo-controlled studies.

Left ventricular performance, measured by radionuclide cineangiography or echocardiography, has been demonstrated to improve with the institution of CEI therapy in some studies. This effect is consistent with a reduction in vasoconstriction and impedance to left ventricular ejection, thus allowing more efficient ventricular emptying and improvement in systolic performance.

CEIs also may benefit renal blood flow. Renal vasodilation may contribute to increases in urinary sodium excretion, which may lead to improvement in sodium and water balance and allow a reduction in the dose of diuretics. Additionally, they may decrease potassium excretion, due to decreased levels of aldosterone, so that the supplementation of potassium-retaining diuretics can be discontinued.

Choice of CEIs

In general, the hemodynamic and neurohormonal effects of CEIs are similar, with the major differences between captopril and enalapril being pharmacokinetic (Table No. 18.1).

Captopril is an active drug, with the onset of hemodynamic effect within 30 minutes after administration, peaking after one to one and one-half hours, and being maintained for a period of six to eight hours.

In contrast, enalapril is a pro drug that must be de-esterified by hepatic esterases to the active form, enalaprilat. It, therefore, has a delayed onset of action to two hours, with a peak effect between four to eight hours, and a long duration of action, with effects persistent for as long as 12 to 24 hours after oral administration.

Such differences indicate that captopril be given on a BID or TID schedule and enalapril on a QD or BID schedule.

Lisinopril, which is not yet FDA-approved for the treatment of heart failure, has an even longer duration of action, which allows it to be given once daily.

Recently, an intravenous formulation of enalapril (the active form, enalaprilat) has been released. This preparation has the same hemodynamic responses as the oral form, with the exception that the onset of action is quite prompt. It produces a marked reduction in systemic vascular resistance and mean arterial pressure within five minutes after administration. Peak response occurs at 30 minutes, with a duration of action as long as 90 minutes.

This preparation may be useful as a pharmacologic probe in investigational studies profiling pathophysiological mechanisms of vasoconstriction in CHF or in clinical situations where the converting enzyme must be blocked rapidly or gastrointestinal absorption is limited.

Side Effects

The seriousness and incidence of side effects with ACE inhibitors are low and represent an acceptable risk in CHF patients in whom the potential benefits are great. These side effects include:

- Taste loss (dysgeusia)
- Skin rash
- Proteinuria
- Neutropenia
- Cough
- Hypotension
- Decreases in renal function

Most of these side effects do not limit drug therapy and are reversible with discontinuation of the drug. In many instances, CEI can be reinstituted without recurrence of the side effect.

The mechanisms of the side effects of ACE inhibitors are complex. It was originally postulated that the sulfhydryl group of captopril was responsible for the side effects, since the symptoms were similar to those seen with penicillamine, another compound containing a sulfhydryl group. However, it has been shown that the side effects seen with enalapril (without the sulfhydryl group) are at least qualitatively similar to captopril. Further studies on the mechanisms of adverse effects are warranted.

Additionally, it has been suggested that the rate of side effects is greater with captopril than with enalapril. However, the data in question were obtained during the use of captopril in high risk patients, such as immunosuppressed patients with collagen vascular diseases, many of whom had evidence of renal dysfunction. Furthermore, the early use of captopril was associated with higher doses of the drug than are currently used. Subsequent studies have shown a decrease in the incidence of side effects with captopril when smaller doses of the drug are used and studied on a larger numbers of patients. Currently, it is not clear whether significant differences between the rates of side effects between captopril and enalapril exist.

Patient Selection

Both captopril and enalapril are FDA-approved for treatment of CHF patients who have not responded adequately to conventional therapy of digitalis and diuretics. Controversy exists about the necessity to maintain digitalis therapy; however, recent data suggest that digoxin is of use in CHF patients, despite its narrow toxic therapeutic ratio (see Section #21).

More recent data from the Digoxin Captopril Trial has suggested that the use of ACE inhibitors is associated with improvements in exercise duration and New York Heart Association classification, as well as decreases in requirements for diuretics, emergency room visits, and hospitalizations for patients with only mild to moderate heart failure (NYHA Class II). Thus, there is a growing trend for initiation of therapy even in patients who do not yet have refractory symptoms. Current studies are being conducted which will assess the use of ACE inhibitors in patients with left ventricular dysfunction who are asymptomatic.

Initiation of Treatment

The most important problem to avoid during the initiation of therapy with ACE inhibitors is hypotension. Since the hemodynamic response is closely correlated with baseline activity of the renin angiotensin system, patients with elevated plasma renin activity may experience a substantial decrease in mean arterial pressure. In these patients, it is advisable to begin therapy at a low dose of 6.25 mg of captopril and to gradually increase the dose to maintenance levels.

If plasma renin activity measurements are not available, clinical correlates allow estimations of that activity (Table 18.2). Patients who are volume depleted, associated with elevations in the BUN/creatinine ratio or the use of large doses of diuretics, generally show high levels of plasma renin activity. Hyponatremia also indicates hyperreninemia. Large reductions in blood pressure may be anticipated in these patients; for them, the initiating dose should be decreased.

Therapy may be initiated under outpatient conditions in reasonably well-compensated patients with normal blood pressures, though the safest procedure is to keep patients under observation for one and one-half hours after administration of the first dose of captopril. Hospitalization may be necessary for patients with borderline (90 to 100 ml systolic) baseline blood pressures or whose adequacy of cardiac reserve is suspect.

Maintenance Therapy

Although diuretic therapy should be continued for the control of edema and elevated cardiac filling pressure, several points should be made about its continued use in patients treated with ACE inhibitors. Because ACE inhibitors decrease levels of aldosterone, thereby decreasing aldosterone-mediated salt and water retention, many patients require lower doses of diuretics. Some patients in whom diuretics are not decreased may develop symptomatic hypotension. Secondly, because of the decrease in aldosterone, potassium levels may increase and the requirement for potassium supplements decrease. Potassium-sparing diuretics (such as spironolactone, amiloride, and triamterene) should be used with caution, since hyperkalemia can occur.

Tachyphylaxis, or the attenuation of beneficial hemodynamic and clinical benefits, is not a significant problem with ACE inhibitors. However, since CHF and the renin angiotensin system are dynamic processes, they are greatly influenced by and dependent upon dietary sodium intake.

A common development with long-term ACE inhibitor use is hypotension. Though this usually occurs within the first 24 hours of initiation therapy, it can occur with long-term treatment, particularly if other vasodilators or diuretics are used.

Hypotension, which can be seen in supine or seated positions or may be orthostatic in nature, can generally be managed by a temporary discontinuation or decrease in the doses of diuretics, ACE inhibitors, or other vasodilators. If extreme volume depletion occurs, volume repletion with oral or intravenous saline may be necessary.

Renal dysfunction is the second most frequent adverse reaction to angiotensin converting inhibitors. On many occasions, renal function improves with the use of ACE inhibitors, likely secondary to an increase in renal plasma flow.

However, patients who experience an excessive reduction of blood pressure or in whom angiotensin-mediated vasoconstriction of the efferent arteriole is critical for maintenance of glomerular filtration rate may develop renal insufficiency with the use of ACE inhibitors. These patients may require a reduction in dosage. In many instances, a temporary reduction in the dose of diuretics, maintaining the dose of the ACE-I, will reverse the renal insufficiency. It cannot be predicted who will develop this response to ACE inhibitors; therefore, follow-up BUN/creatinine is recommended when ACE inhibitor therapy is begun.

TABLE 18.1 – **Pharmacokinetic Differences Between Captopril and Enalapril**

	Captopril	**Enalapril**
Oral absorption	60 to 75%	60 to 75%
Excretion	Renal	Renal
Onset	15 to 30 minutes	2 to 4 hours
Peak	60 to 90 minutes	4 to 8 hours
Duration	6 to 8 hours	12 to 24 hours

TABLE 18.2 – **Correlates of Increased Plasma Renin Activity**

- Volume depletion
- Increase BUN/creatinine ratio
- Hyponatremia
- Intensive diuretic therapy

#19 Digitalis: Indications and Contraindications

Digitalis was discovered in the late 1700s by William Withering and has long been one of the mainstays of CHF treatment. Its mechanism of action is the inhibition of the sodium-potassium ATPase in myocardial cells, which leads to an increase in intracellular sodium. This leads to an increase in intracellular calcium through the sodium-calcium exchange mechanism, and the resulting increased availability of intracellular calcium to the contractile proteins leads to an increase in the contractile force. This inotropic effect is manifested by an upward and leftward shift of the ventricular function curve so that, at any given ventricular filling pressure, there is an increase in stroke work.

Digitalis may contribute to patients' arrhythmia problems, since it also:

- Increases the duration of action potential
- Increases Phase IV depolarization
- Reduces resting membrane potential

The clinical efficacy of digitalis in CHF patients has been somewhat controversial. Although it effectively controls the ventricular rate in patients with atrial fibrillation, its efficacy as an inotropic agent and its value in patients with normal sinus rhythm has been debated. However, it is now generally agreed that digitalis leads to sustained improvement in cardiac function, using invasive hemodynamics, non-invasive assessments of left ventricular function, and other clinical parameters. Thus, the clinical utility of digoxin has been affirmed for patients with mild or moderate symptoms of heart failure.

Appropriate patient selection is necessary, since the efficacy of digitalis is less well-substantiated for patients with hypertrophied or non-dilated hearts or for those with left ventricular dysfunction but no symptoms of heart failure.

19.

Furthermore, recent data in prospective, randomized, placebo-controlled, double-blind trials in CHF patients have confirmed the efficacy of digitalis. In the Digoxin Captopril Trials, for example, when compared to placebo, digoxin was associated with:

- An increase in ejection fraction by nuclear scanning
- A decreased need for diuretics
- A decreased need for hospital admissions and emergency room visits

In a milrinone (an experimental inotropic agent) trial, patients randomized to digoxin showed significant improvement in exercise duration during treadmill testing.

Although new studies confirm the indication of digitalis for the early treatment of CHF patients, possible risks with digitalis therapy, because of its potential arrhythmogenic effect, have not been addressed in an appropriate study.

#20 Pharmacokinetics of Digitalis Preparations/Clinical Use

Pharmacokinetics

Two digitalis preparations are available for CHF patients:

- Digitoxin
- Digoxin

The main difference between the two are their pharmacokinetics, as summarized in Table 20.1.

Digitoxin

Digitoxin, the non-polar form, is almost completely absorbed from the gastrointestinal tract. It is avidly bound to serum proteins and is excreted by the liver after metabolic degradation. Thus, while digitoxin doses do not have to be significantly changed in patients with renal insufficiency, doses must be decreased in patients with significant degrees of liver failure.

The half-life of digitoxin is prolonged to five to seven days, giving it the advantages of:

- Infrequent dosing
- No profound adverse effects if a dose is missed

In clinical practice, however, digitoxin is less frequently used than digoxin because of the difficulties associated with:

- Titrating dosages
- Its long half-life (for patients with digitalis toxicity)

Digoxin

Most physicians prescribe digoxin for their CHF patients because it is reasonably well absorbed and is excreted unchanged in the kidney. Doses must be decreased in patients with renal insufficiency, which is a common occurrence in CHF patients.

A relatively recent delivery system of digoxin is the gelatin capsule, which has increased the absorption bioavailability of digoxin to 90 to 100 percent. Consequently, the normal maintenance dose is approximately 20 percent less than that of digoxin in the tablet form (0.1 to 0.2 mg per day).

Clinical Use

Many CHF patients are given a full digitalizing dose in order to rapidly achieve steady state drug levels and the full drug benefit. The average digitalizing dosages are:

- For digitoxin - Approximately 1 mg
- For digoxin - Between 1 and 1.5 mg

Digitalizing doses can be given orally or intravenously, depending on the clinical urgency necessary to achieve steady state levels, and they are generally given in divided doses over a 24-hour period. It is also possible to initiate a maintenance dose of digoxin or digitoxin (without a loading dose) that will eventually result in adequate digitalization.

The clinical use of digitalis is somewhat complicated by the lack of an easily identifiable end point assessing therapeutic efficacy. Given the considerable risk of digitalis toxicity (see Section #21), it is generally not advisable to "push" doses of digitalis to maximally-tolerated limits. Thus, the digitalizing dose is commonly followed by a daily maintenance dose, based on the patient's size, gender, and renal function.

The absorption and excretion rates of digitalis are variable, as are individual sensitivities to its cardiac effect. When there is concern about the adequacy or safety of a dose of digoxin, blood levels should be measured.

TABLE 20.1 – **Pharmacokinetics of Digitalis Preparations**

	Digitoxin	**Digoxin**
Oral absorption	90 to 100%	50 to 75%
Excretion route	Liver and metabolites	Renal and unchanged
T 1/2	5 to 7 days	1.5 days
Maintenance dose	0.1 to 0.15 mg	0.125 to 0.25 mg

#21 Digitalis Toxicity

Despite its clinical efficacy, the use of digitalis is associated with adverse reactions due to its narrow toxic-to-therapeutic ratio. Although the incidence of adverse effects has decreased in recent years, digitalis toxicity still accounts for a number of potential serious complications. Tables 21.1 and 21.2 list some of the more common extra-cardiac and cardiac manifestations of digitalis toxicity.

Digitalis has been known to cause almost every known arrhythmia and may, in fact, result in death. Important to the diagnosis of early digitalis toxicity are the electrocardiogram and close monitoring of digoxin levels in the patient. However, patients showing "therapeutic levels" of digoxin can demonstrate toxicity, while patients showing "toxic levels" may not demonstrate any of its signs. This phenomenon may be of particular importance for patients with atrial fibrillation whose digitalis levels are a less reliable indication of toxicity. Additionally, no "classic" electrocardiographic signs exist to distinguish digitalis toxicity from spontaneously-occurring arrhythmias.

Several types of patients are particularly at risk for developing digitalis toxicity (Table 21.3). Elderly patients and those with renal insufficiency have a decreased ability to excrete digoxin and so may accumulate toxic levels.

In hypothyroidism, drug levels are also increased, due to a prolongation of the elimination half-life. In hyperthyroidism, digoxin elimination is increased and end organ resistance to the drug's effect is possible.

Hypoxia and several metabolic abnormalities, including hypokalemia and hypomagnesemia may also accentuate digitalis toxicity. Such metabolic abnormalities are common in CHF patients, either as a direct result of heart dysfunction or as an effect of drug therapy (especially diuretics), and, thus, the monitoring of serum levels of potassium and magnesium in these patients is critical.

Additionally, metabolism and excretion of digoxin are affected by the large number of drugs which CHF patients may take. Quinidine, for example, decreases the volume of distribution of digoxin and reduces renal clearance of it, resulting in increased levels. Similar effects have been reported with verapamil and amiodarone. In these cases, digoxin dosages should be decreased to avoid toxicity.

Management of Toxicity

Initially, management of patients with digitalis toxicity should include:

- Stopping the administration of digoxin
- Monitoring digoxin levels
- Performing an electrocardiogram

This routine is effective in most cases of digitalis toxicity, and, given its half-life of 36 hours, levels should decrease in one to two days, assuming renal function is normal. This is the most appropriate therapy for patients who are stable hemodynamically and clinically.

A patient may be compromised with ventricular tachycardia or junctional arrhythmias, however, as manifest by a decrease in:

- Blood pressure
- Urine output
- Level of consciousness

In this case, the initial step is to reverse the confounding influences, such as hypoxia and/or metabolic abnormalities. Lidocaine is frequently useful to control ventricular ectopic rhythms, though it is not useful in junctional tachycardia. Phenytoin is also effective.

Cardioversion is useful for patients with life-threatening arrhythmias, though it is not generally recommended because of the high incidence of arrhythmias following cardioversion.

Recently, digoxin-specific antibodies have been approved for serious digitalis toxicity and are available in most hospital formularies. These antibodies are effective in reversing the clinical toxicity of digitalis excess.

TABLE 21.1 — **Extra Cardiac Manifestations of Digitalis Toxicity**

1. Anorexia
2. Nausea, vomiting
3. Fatigue and weakness
4. Visual disturbances
5. Confusion, disorientation
6. Hallucinations

TABLE 21.2 — **Cardiac Manifestations of Digitalis Toxicity**

1. Ventricular premature contractions
2. Atrioventricular nodal rhythm
3. Paroxysmal atrial tachycardia with AV block
4. Sinus arrest or sinoatrial exit block
5. Second degree AV block (Mobitz I)
6. Low ventricular rate with atrial fibrillation

TABLE 21.3 — **Patients at Risk for Digitalis Toxicity**

1. Elderly
2. Renal insufficiency
3. Hypothyroidism
4. Hypoxia
5. Metabolic abnormalities
6. Drug interactions

#22 Beta Blockers

Although treatment of CHF patients who have systolic dysfunction with agents having potent negative inotropic effects (such as a beta blockers) appears counterintuitive, recent data suggest that this form of drug therapy may be beneficial for long-term treatment. In an uncontrolled study of 46 patients with dilated cardiomyopathy, three-year survival was increased in patients receiving beta blockers, as compared to controls; drug withdrawal, in those demonstrating clinical improvement while on beta blockers, was associated with patients' significant deterioration. Additionally, in a randomized, double-blind, placebo-controlled trial, patients receiving metoprolol showed a significant improvement in exercise capacity, functional class, and ejection fraction.

The mechanisms by which beta blocking therapy may be of long-term benefit are unknown but may involve:

- The antagonism of the increased sympathetic tone typical of CHF patients
- Anti-ischemic effects
- Anti-arrhythmic effects

More recent data has shown that chronic sympathetic stimulation leads to a reduction in beta-receptor sites and reduced responsiveness to catecholamine stimulation. Beta blockers may reverse this "down regulation" and restore the response of the heart to adrenergic stimulation.

Despite the provocative nature of these initial reports, the use of beta blockers is still considered experimental and cannot be applied as standard therapy for CHF patients. These initial studies involved small numbers of patients, and many of these patients were excluded from the results because of their intolerance to beta blocker therapy. The beneficial effects of beta blockers must be confirmed in randomized, controlled studies involving large patient populations before its use can be universally sanctioned.

22.

#23 Experimental Inotropic Agents

Since many patients with severe CHF remain symptomatic despite digitalis and vasodilator therapy, researchers are intensively seeking an orally-active inotropic agent which will:

- Stimulate cardiac contractility
- Improve hemodynamic profiles of patients
- Improve the clinical status of patients
- Have no significant adverse effects

Prototypes for the development of such inotropic agents are the two beta-adrenergic agonists:

- Dopamine
- Dobutamine

These agents are effective for use in intensive care but are limited for long-term use because:

- They must be administered intravenously
- They may be associated with tachyphylaxis (see Sections #18 and #19)

Under investigation are several different types of orally-active agents, including:

- Beta-adrenergic agonists
- Phosphodiesterase inhibitors
- Other membrane channel drugs

Several orally-active beta-agonists, including pirbuterol and prenaterol, have been studied, but despite their demonstration of initial improvement in hemodynamics of CHF patients, long-term administration has been limited due to chronotropic effects.

The phosphodiesterase inhibitors inhibit the degradation of cyclic AMP; subsequent increased intracellular cyclic AMP concentrations activate protein kinases that lead to:

- Increased calcium delivery to the contractile proteins
- A positive inotropic effect

The phosphodiesterase inhibitors that have been evaluated include:

- Amrinone – Now FDA-approved as an intravenous preparation (see Sections #18 and #19); no oral preparation is available for chronic administration
- Milrinone – Also FDA-approved for intravenous administration. However, trials to assess long-term benefits with the oral formulation have recently been discontinued
- Enoximone – Also in Phase III clinical trials

23.

Recently, newer agents which do not act directly on the beta-receptor complex or concentrations of cyclic AMP have been investigated. These drugs, such as OPC-8212 and pimobendan, may sensitize contractile proteins to calcium or increase intracellular sodium concentration, thereby leading to an increase in calcium by the sodium-calcium exchange mechanism and avoiding adverse effects associated with the phosphodiesterase inhibitors. Additional data are necessary, however, to assess efficacy of these agents.

#24 General Considerations

CHF patients are generally admitted or transferred to intensive care units when the following conditions or complications occur:

- Pulmonary edema
- Severe hypotension and shock
- Signs and symptoms of heart failure refractory to intensive oral medications
- Need for close monitoring of arrhythmias

The initial assessment and management of the severely decompensated CHF patient is the same as that for a patient of any medical emergency. Assessment should include an evaluation of the adequacy of:

- Airway
- Breathing
- Circulation

An adequate airway must be secured. Intubation may be required with severe pulmonary edema if massive amounts of alveolar fluid prevent adequate ventilation and oxygenation.

It is usually important to obtain an arterial blood gas in order to:

- Measure the adequacy of oxygenation
- Ascertain the need for supplemental oxygen therapy
- Gain information regarding acid base balance, including:
    - pCO_2
    - Possible metabolic acidosis due to circulatory insufficiency

The adequacy of circulation can be quickly assessed by examining patients with particular reference to:

- Blood pressure
- Level of alertness
- Urine output
- Character of extremities and peripheral pulses

Patients who have decompensated heart failure and pulmonary edema may still have sufficient "forward flow" or perfusion of vital organ beds, as manifested by acceptable:

- Blood pressure (greater than 90 systolic)
- Urine output (greater than 20 cc per hour)
- Peripheral pulse amplitude

In contrast, patients who develop circulatory insufficiency will have:

- Hypotension (systolic blood pressure less than 90 mm Hg)
- Signs of acute peripheral vasoconstriction
- Weak and thready pulses
- Cool, cyanotic extremities

In the most severe cases, patients may:

- Become lethargic
- Become stuporous
- Have gradually decreasing urine output
- Experience acute tubular necrosis with anuria

These patients require invasive monitoring (see Section #27).

The preliminary evaluation should also include an investigation of potential causes of decompensation of heart failure (see Section #2). Acute pulmonary edema can occur without preexisting ventricular dysfunction (such as in acute myocardial infarction) with a ventricular septal defect or papillary muscle dysfunction. In some instances, acute pulmonary edema can be the initial presenting sign of critical mitral stenosis or myocardial ischemia (angina or silent). Therefore, the evaluation of potential causes must be thorough and comprehensive.

Additionally, the initial evaluation should include:

- Electrocardiogram
- Chest x-ray
- Complete blood count
- Electrolyte analysis
- Urinalysis
- Liver function tests
- Blood/urine cultures, if infection is suspected

The electrocardiogram may give important information concerning the presence of myocardial ischemia/infarction or arrhythmias, both of which may be underlying precipitating factors in patients with pulmonary edema.

The chest x-ray may indicate the signs of:

- Infiltrates
- Pleural effusions
- Pulmonary vascular redistribution

The lag period should be taken into consideration of assessment, since typical roentgenographic findings of pulmonary edema lag behind classic physical findings and their resolutions by up to several days.

The white blood cell count can be evaluated during any time of stress. Profound anemia can precipitate decompensations of heart failure.

The electrolyte analysis and urinalysis are important guides concerning:

- Acid base and metabolic balance
- Adequacy of renal function

#25 Patterns of Hemodynamic Instability

Patients should undergo invasive, bedside, hemodynamic monitoring with indwelling right heart catheters if they:

- Do not respond to typical treatment interventions
- Display signs of profound circulatory insufficiency (see Sections #11 and #26)

In these situations, patients may need to be transferred to tertiary care hospitals where personnel experienced in the use of these catheters are available.

The catheters are inserted via the internal jugular, subclavian, or antecubital vein and are then advanced through the right atrium and right ventricle to assess right and left heart filling pressures ("preload"), including:

- Right atrial (RA)
- Pulmonary artery systolic (PAS)
- Pulmonary artery diastolic (PAD)
- Pulmonary capillary wedge pressures (PWP)

Cardiac output is also monitored via thermodilution computers.

General Patterns of Instability
High PA/PCW Pressures

Hemodynamic instability occurs in three general patterns, as outlined in Table 25.1. The first column of the table outlines the pattern characterized chiefly by the marked elevation in cardiac filling pressures with increases in right atrial, pulmonary artery, and pulmonary wedge pressures. In this case, the systemic arterial pressure is adequate, and, although cardiac output is decreased, it is not severely depressed.

Patients with this pattern are best treated with interventions that decrease preload and pulmonary congestion, including diuretic agents. In addition, the use of vasodilating agents could further decrease preload via venodilation and increase cardiac output via decreases in afterload and impedance (see Section #3).

Low Cardiac Output

The second column of Table 25.1 outlines profiles in which patients have marked elevations in preload and cardiac filling pressures but also have marked reductions in cardiac output and systemic blood pressures.

These patients may require treatment with diuretics and vasodilators. However, since such treatment may be limited by further decreases in blood pressure, the introduction of inotropic agents may be of some benefit.

Low Blood Pressure

The third column of the table outlines the primary hemodynamic problem of a profound reduction in systemic arterial pressure. These patients are critically ill and require vasopressor agents for circulatory support.

TABLE 25.1 — **Patterns of Hemodynamic Instability**

	I. High PA/PCW Pressures	II. Low Cardiac Output	III. Low Blood Pressure
RA	20	20	15
PA	65/40	65/40	50/30
PWP	37	37	25
AP	110/70	90/70	60/40
CO	3.70	2.50	2.50
RX	Diuretics and Vasodilators	Inotropic Agents	Vasopressors

NOTES

#26 Drug Treatment

Vasodilators

Although orally adminstered vasodilators can be given to patients with hemodynamic instability, it is generally preferable to use parenterally administered vasodilators to:

- Achieve more precisely titrated dosages and hemodynamic responses
- Gain an ability to rapidly decrease dosages, e.g. in case of excessive hypotension
- Eliminate the possibility of difficulties associated with incomplete oral absorption

The two commonly-used vasodilators in the management of acutely ill patients with heart failure are:

- Nitroprusside
- Nitroglycerin

Nitroprusside

Nitroprusside is one of the most potent dilators. Important guidelines concerning its use are summarized in Table 26.1.

Nitroprusside offers a balanced action of venous capacitance vessels and arterial resistance vessels, thereby lowering:

- Preload
- The signs and symptoms of pulmonary congestion
- Afterload/impedance

The vasodilator action leads to increases in cardiac output even in patients with borderline low blood pressure.

The dose of nitroprusside is titrated against the desired hemodynamic effect. This will usually involve:

- A reduction in pulmonary capillary wedge or pulmonary artery diastolic pressure to 15 to 20 mm Hg
- An increase in cardiac output that maintains cerebral, renal, and myocardial perfusion (generally above 4 to 5 L/min)

Since the desired effect and dose response relationship varies according to the severity of the decompensation and the concomitant pharmacologic therapy, it is important to monitor the:

- Overall hemodynamic profile
- Changes brought about by each infusion rate of nitroprusside

Hypotension, the principal adverse reaction to nitroprusside, actually represents a pharmacologic action of this potent vasodilator. In such a case, therapy should be adjusted to:

- Decrease the dose of nitroprusside
- Decrease the use of diuretics
- Decrease the use of drugs with vasodilatory actions
- Consider the institution of inotropic drug support

Thiocyanate poisoning can develop, especially in patients given prolonged infusions of nitroprusside or with concomitant renal insufficiency.

Nitroglycerin

Nitroglycerin can be administered parenterally to patients with decompensated CHF and may be especially helpful for patients with coronary artery disease who are deteriorating because of ongoing myocardial ischemia. In contrast to nitroprusside, nitroglycerin has a more predominant effect on venous capacitance vessels, thus causing a greater reduction in preload and a smaller effect on afterload.

Nitroglycerin must be carefully titrated against the desired hemodynamic effect. Its primary adverse reaction, as with any vasodilator, is hypotension, an effect which reflects its predominant pharmacologic action. Because the diluent contains ethanol, alcohol intoxication has been reported in patients receiving prolonged infusion of nitroglycerin.

Inotropic Agents

Four inotropic agents that are available for intravenous treatment of patients with decompensated CHF and inadequate cardiac output are:

- Dopamine
- Dobutamine
- Amrinone
- Milrinone

Tables 26.3 through 26.5 list the general features of these agents.

Dopamine

Dopamine, which has an important dose/response relationship, is one of the most commonly used drugs for intensive care unit patients.

At low doses (less than 4ug/kg/min), dopamine appears to act preferentially on dopaminergic receptors, especially in the renal vasculature. This may improve renal blood flow and promote a natriuresis in the absence of a systemic effect on cardiac output or blood pressure.

At slightly higher doses (between 4 to 8 ug/kg/min), dopamine stimulates beta-receptors, with subsequent increases in contractility and heart rate, leading to improvement in cardiac output.

At higher doses (> 8 ug/kg/min), dopamine stimulates alpha-receptors in the peripheral vasculature, causing vasoconstriction and thereby maintaining blood pressure.

With careful titration of dosages, several different effects of this drug may be elicited. Its most common use is as adjunct therapy, given in the dopaminergic range.

Dobutamine

Dobutamine is the intravenous sympathomimetic agent which comes closest to providing a specific inotropic effect by selectively increasing contractility. This effect can be provided without altering the patient's heart rate or blood pressure because of the drug's specific beta1-receptor activity.

Dobutamine has several advantages over dopamine (Table 26.4):

- It does not tend to increase heart rate unless doses are increased to more than 7 ug/kg/min
- It has less effect on alpha-adrenergic receptors and peripheral vasculature and, therefore, will not increase peripheral vasoconstriction
- When compared to beta-stimulation from dopamine, it appears to cause a greater decrease in preload, manifested by:
  - Larger reductions in pulmonary artery pressure
  - Larger reductions in pulmonary capillary wedge pressure
- It causes a smaller increase in myocardial oxygen consumption

Given these considerations, dobutamine appears to be the inotropic drug of choice in patients with decompensated heart failure.

The dose of dobutamine must be titrated against the specific desired hemodynamic effect. The initial dose is typically between 2 to 5 ug/kg/min, titrated against:

- Cardiac output
- Pulmonary artery and pulmonary wedge pressures
- Clinical indications of adequate circulation

Using these parameters, the dose can be increased to a maximum of approximately 20 ug/kg/min. Although such doses can be maintained for long periods of time, prolonged use is a concern because:

- Its beneficial effects may tend to attenuate
- It may provoke ventricular arrhythmias

It is important to note that additive effects can be obtained when combining dobutamine with a vasodilator such as nitroprusside.

Amrinone

Amrinone is a bipyridine compound whose mechanism of action involves its activity as a phosphodiesterase inhibitor. It does not appear to have any activity on adrenergic receptors or sodium potassium ATPase. In addition to augmenting contractility, amrinone is a potent peripheral vasodilator, so that its hemodynamic profile is characterized by:

- An increase in cardiac output
- A decrease in pulmonary artery pressure
- A decrease in systemic vascular resistance

In some studies, amrinone has been demonstrated to actually decrease myocardial oxygen consumption, presumably because the reduction in wall tension is greater than the effect on the increase in contractility.

Amrinone is generally given as a bolus of 0.5 to 1 mg/kg, followed by a sustaining infusion of 5 to 10 ug/kg/min. If the desired hemodynamic effect becomes attenuated following the bolus, an additional bolus of 0.5 to 1 mg/kg can be given, with a maximum dose of about 10 mg/kg/day.

Potential adverse effects of this drug are a concern, although accurate evaluations have been difficult to obtain because of the severity of patients' illnesses. Thrombocytopenia, at an incidence of approximately two to four percent, has been known to complicate amrinone therapy, and gastointestinal discomfort and liver function abnormalities have been noted in a small percentage of patients. As with any inotropic agent, the provocation of atrial and ventricular arrhymias are of major concern.

Vasopressor Agents

When the hemodynamic profile of patients with decompensated heart failure is characterized by hypotension, specific measures must be instituted to support circulation, so that the mean arterial pressure is kept above 65 to 70 mmHg in order to maintain the adequacy of cerebral, renal, and cardiac circulations. The prognosis of these patients is extremely poor.

To fully understand the hemodynamic profile of the sympathomimetic agents available for use as vasopressor support, it is necessary to review their effects on alpha- and beta-receptors, summarized in Table 26.6. Stimulation of alpha-receptors in the peripheral vasculature causes vasoconstriction, stimulation of beta1-cardiac receptors causes increases in heart rate and contractility, and stimulation of beta2-receptors in the peripheral vasculature subserves vasodilation.

Norepinephrine has strong stimulatory effects on alpha-peripheral receptors, causing vasoconstriction. In addition, it has potent effects on beta1-cardiac receptors to increase heart rate and cardiac output.

Epinephrine has similar effects to norephinephrine. However, it also has some beta2 activity so that the vasopressor effect is less pronounced than that of norephinephrine.

Isoproterenol has no activity on alpha-receptors but is a potent stimulant of both beta1- and beta2-receptors. Therefore, although it is effective in increasing cardiac output and heart rate, it is relatively ineffective in increasing blood pressure in patients with profound hypotension.

Phenylephrine is a potent alpha-receptor stimulant and so will cause vasoconstriction. It has no effect on beta-receptors, however, and will not cause an increase in contractility or heart rate. It will, in fact, generally lead to cardiac slowing due to autonomic nervous system reflexes activated by the increase in blood pressure.

Dopamine has specific dose-related activities on alpha- and beta-receptors and can be used to help support circulation in high doses.

Dobutamine, because it has less effect on alpha-receptors on the peripheral vasculature, is less useful as a single agent when severe hypotension exists.

The most commonly used sympathomimetic amine in the treatment of patients with profound hypotension is norepinephrine. The exact dose is variable, based on the severity of the reduction in blood pressure and of left ventricular dysfunction. Generally, it is started at a dose of 1 to 2 ug/min, with close titration of blood pressure, and is gradually increased until the mean arterial pressure is in the range of 60 to 70 mm Hg. When the mean arterial pressure is increased above these levels, additional peripheral vasoconstriction may further depress myocardial performance by contributing to excessive impedance and may also lead to a critical reduction in renal blood flow because of intense renal vasoconstriction. These characterics also apply to the use of epinephrine.

Given the potency of this sympathomimetic agonist, significant side effects are anticipated. This drug causes a dose-related positive chronotropic effect and a marked increase in heart rate, which may lead to atrial and ventricular arrhythmias.

TABLE 26.1 – **Nitroprusside**

Initial Dose	0.1 ug/kg/min = 5 to 10 ug/min
Increased By	0.1 to 0.3 ug/kg/min - 5 to 10 ug/min
Titrate To	PA/PCW/CO
Adverse Effects	Hypotension, cyanide poisoning

TABLE 26.2 – **Nitroglycerin**

Initial Dose	5 to 10 ug/min
Increased By	5 to 10 ug/min
Titrate To	PA/PCW/CO
Adverse Effects	Hypotension, alcohol intoxication

TABLE 26.3 – **Dopamine**

Dopaminergic	Less than 4ug/kg/min
Beta	4 to 8 ug/kg/min
Alpha	> 8 ug/kg/min
Advantages	Dopaminergic increases RBF Can support blood pressure

TABLE 26.4 – **Dobutamine**

Advantages of Dobutamine

- Does not increase HR
- Less effect on alpha receptors (BP)
- Greater decrease in PA/PCW
- Less increase in MVO2
- Dose:
    - Initial 5 ug/kg/min
    - Titer CO/PA/PWP
    - Maximum 20 ug/kg/min

TABLE 26.5 – **Amrinone (Inocor®)**

Class:	Bipyridine
Mechanism:	Phosphodiesterase inhibitor
Actions:	Increases contractility
	Decreases PWP and MVO2
Bolus:	0.75 mg/kg
Infusion:	5 to 10 ug/kg/min
Additional Bolus:	0.75 mg/kg
Maximum Dose:	10 mg/kg/day
Adverse Effects:	Thrombocytopenia (2 to 4%) GI (1 to 2%) Arrhythmia (3%) Liver (1 to 2%)

TABLE 26.6 – **Sympathomimetic Amines**

	Alpha Peripheral (Vasoconstriction)	B-1 Cardiac (HR/SV)	B-2 Peripheral (Vasodilation)
Norepinephrine	++++	+++	0
Epinephrine	++++	++++	++
Isoproterenol	0	++++	++++
Phenylephrine	++++	0	0
Dopamine*	++	++++	++
Dobutamine	+	++++	++

*Also has dopaminergic activity

Norepinephrine

Indication: Hypotension

Dose: 2 to 8 ug/min

Titrate To: MAP 60 to 70 mmHg – If MAP is greater than 70, may decrease perfusion

Adverse Effects: Tachycardia
Arrhythmias
Nonspecific vasoconstriction

NOTES

#27 Devices

Mechanical interventions should be considered for patients with profound circulatory collapse that is unresponsive to potent inotropic and vasopressor vasodilator agents (Table 27.1). This will require patient transfer to tertiary care hospitals where cardiac surgery is available. The common mechanical devices include:

- Intra-aortic balloon pump (IABP)
- Left ventricular assist device (LVAD)
- Artificial heart
- Emergent cardiac transplantation (see Section #28)

Intra-Aortic Balloon Pump

The intra-aortic balloon pump (Table 27.2) assists circulation and provides hemodynamic stabilization. Its action:

- Reduces afterload
- Increases cardiac output by 20 to 30 percent
- Augments diastolic blood pressure
- Improves coronary perfusion

The advantage of the balloon pump is that it can be inserted rapidly and percutaneously for prompt stabilization of circulation. It is most commonly employed when the cause for deterioration in hemodynamics is reversible, since it provides temporary stabilization until a more definitive therapy can be performed, e.g., coronary artery bypass surgery. If the reversible cause is acute decompensation associated with arrhythmias or infections, antiarrhythmic therapy and/or antibiotics will likely improve patients' overall condition.

The IABP is not usually used in cases of end-stage heart failure in which no reversible process can be identified or in which no additional therapy is anticipated.

Risks of infection and bleeding are present with long-term use of the IABP, because of the catheter's large size and of the requirement for systemic heparinization used to prevent thrombosis. Thrombocytopenia risk is also substantial. Additionally, the placement of the large catheter in the femoral artery can compromise circulation to the leg, especially in patients with peripheral vascular disease.

The timing of inflation and deflation of the balloon is set against patients' heart rhythm and the recognition of the QRS complex on the electrocardiogram. It is therefore anticipated that balloon pumping is less efficient with both atrial and ventricular arrhythmias or where there is marked irregularity of heart rhythm.

Left Ventricular Assist Device/Artificial Heart

The left ventricular assist device (LVAD) and the artificial heart are two recent mechanical devices designed to assist circulation in extraordinary cases. Both continue to undergo refinement.

These devices require major cardiac surgery for implantation and are considered to be only temporary treatment measures for patients in whom cardiac transplantation is expected. In most cases, the maximum period of time that the LVAD may remain implanted is 10 to 15 days. After their implantation, cardiac transplantation is more difficult because of increased risks of:

- Infection
- Thrombosis
- Hemorrhage

Of the two devices, the LVAD is the current treatment of choice when the IABP is insufficient. Although it does require a sternotomy and places the patient at high infection risk because of the required tubes leading from the heart to the external pump, the LVAD has proven to stabilize patients until an appropriate donor heart can be obtained.

The same procedure is usually adopted for implantation of the total artificial heart. This device is currently investigational and may have a higher incidence of infections, hemotysis, and thromboembolism. These problems will likely be minimized in the future via refinement of the device.

Total heart replacement eliminates the possibility that the native heart may recover function.

TABLE 27.1 – **Additional Measures in Refractory CHF**

1. IABP
2. LVAD
3. Artificial heart
4. Cardiac transplantation

TABLE 27.2 – **Intra-Aortic Balloon Pump**

Indications:

Hemodynamic stabilization for a reversible process

Actions:

Increase CO 20 to 30 percent
Increase diastolic BP
Increase coronary blood flow

Problems:

Infection
Bleeding
Thrombocytopenia
Leg ischemia
Less effective with arrhythmias

#28 Transplantation

General

Cardiac transplantation remains one of the most dramatic and successful interventions for patients with severe, intractable CHF. While the survival of patients with end-stage heart failure is poor, with two-year survival rates of approximately 30 to 50 percent (see Section #8), the survival of a comparable group of patients undergoing cardiac transplantation is 80 to 90 percent at one-year in most centers. Additionally, the majority of transplant patients lead active lives, many being able to return to full employment and enjoying many activities which were severely limited prior to transplantation.

Cardiac transplantation is no longer considered an experimental or investigational procedure but the next logical treatment for patients with end-stage heart failure.

Indications

Table 28.1 lists the most common indications for cardiac transplantation, with symptoms of heart failure that are refractory to intensive medication regimens being the most common.

Category I

Patients in this first category are generally treated with:

- Salt restriction
- Digitalis
- Large doses of diuretics
- Vasodilators (see Sections #17 through #20)

They usually continue to have such disabling symptoms as dyspnea, exercise intolerance, and fatigue, and therapy via pharmacologic interventions cannot usually be advanced because of:

- Drug toxicity
- Excessive hypotension
- Increases in renal insufficiency

Category II

Patients with intractable angina pectoris are considered candidates for cardiac transplantation, even if they do not experience symptoms typically associated with CHF. These patients have profound exercise intolerance due primarily to angina or myocardial ischemia.

Although these patients are commonly referred for coronary artery bypass surgery, a certain subset of these patients do not have coronary anatomy suitable for standard bypass surgery and/or percutaneous transluminal coronary angioplasty. This occurs often in patients with:

- Diffuse atherosclerotic disease
- Poor distal filling
- High grade stenosis in relatively small coronary vessels

Although many of these patients respond to intensive anti-anginal medication, including high doses of nitrates, calcium channel blockers, and the judicious use of beta blockers, many continue to have symptoms of angina that limit the activities of daily life. Thus, they are considered candidates for cardiac transplantation.

Category III

Those patients with recurrent ventricular arrhythmias and/or sudden cardiac death are also candidates for transplantation. The majority of these patients have undergone extensive electrophysiologic testing and multiple anti-arrhythmic drug trials, and many patients are controlled by the automatic implantable cardioverter but require frequent shocks, suggesting that they are at high risk for sudden cardiac death.

Despite these measures, some patients continue to have significant ventricular arrhythmias and episodes of sudden cardiac death and are considered for transplantation even in the absence of significant signs and symptoms of heart failure.

As cardiac transplantation success continues to increase, indications for the procedure may also be modified. It can be anticipated, therefore, that other conditions might be considered indications for transplantation in the future. However, limitation of donor supply will continue to restrict the numbers of heart transplants performed.

Exclusions

Age

Table 28.2 lists the generally accepted exclusion criteria for cardiac transplantation. Many transplant centers currently consider patients up to the age of 65 years as transplant candidates, since the success of patients in this age group appears to be similar to that of younger patients. However, this experience is not uniform, especially in view of the morbidity rates related to immunosuppressant medications; in many centers the upper age limit is still 55 years. Furthermore, many centers have used the lower age limit because of the continuing shortage of donor organs.

Pulmonary Complications

Patients with marked elevations in pulmonary vascular resistance and "fixed" pulmonary hypertension are at high risk for post-operative complications of transplant surgery, including ventilator dependence and right ventricular dysfunction. Therefore, patients will not be considered for transplantation if:

- The pulmonary vascular resistance is greater than 6 Wood units (480 d.s.cm-5)
- Pulmonary pressures are unresponsive to the administration of potent vasodilators, e.g., nitroprusside

Disease

Patients with concomitant diseases incur substantially increased risks of post-operative complications, such as renal insufficiency and opportunistic infection. Therefore, patients with abnormalities whose severity is out of the typical range associated with heart failure are not optimal candidates for transplantation.

Abnormalities likely to exclude cardiac transplantation include:

- Hepatic dysfunction – Total bilirubin greater than 1.5 to 2.0 mg/dl

- Renal insufficiency :
  - Serum creatinine greater than 1.5 mg/dl
    – or –
  - Creatinine clearance less than 50 ml/min
- Pulmonary dysfunction – FEV1 less than 50 percent predicted on DLCO less than 50 percent predicted
- Uncontrolled diabetes mellitus, complicated by:
  - Retinopathy
  - Nephropathy
  - Vascular disease

Similarly, patients with recent (less than six weeks) pulmonary embolism are at high risk for pulmonary infections in the immediate post-operative period. Patients with bleeding diatheses or gastrointestinal bleeding due to peptic ulcer disease have a high incidence of bleeding post-operatively and are therefore treated and controlled prior to transplantation.

Currently, concern about long-term effects of immunosuppressant therapy on development neoplastic disorders, such as lymphoma, with regard to transplantation has increased. Patients with histories of malignancy will likely be excluded, therefore, unless a cure is demonstrated, as with certain basal cell carcinomas.

TABLE 28.1 – **Indications for Cardiac Transplantation**

1. Severe Class III-IV heart failure – Unresponsive to an intensive medication regimen
2. Intractable angina pectoris
3. Recurrent ventricular arrhymias and/or sudden cardiac death

TABLE 28.2 – **Exclusion Criteria for Cardiac Transplantation**

1. Age greater than 65 years
2. Pulmonary vascular resistance greater than 6 Wood units
3. Irreversible hepatic, renal or pulmonary dysfunction
4. Uncontrolled or complicated diabetes mellitus
5. Active infection
6. Recent pulmonary embolism
7. Bleeding diathesis
8. GI bleeding
9. Malignancy

#29 Complications of Cardiac Transplantation

The most common complaints of cardiac transplantation are listed in Table 29.1. Acute cardiac rejection may manifest itself in various ways. Severe cases are characterized by cardiac failure with:

- Congestive symptoms
- Decreasing blood pressure
- Decreasing cardiac output
- Arrhythmias

With the advances and refinements in the immunosuppressant protocol, acute rejection culminating in cardiac failure is relatively uncommon today. The introduction of cyclosporine in the 1980s to the immunosuppressant protocol is probably one of the more important factors contributing to the prevention of acute transplant rejection. Today, most rejections are clinically silent and are detected via routine endomyocardial biopsies.

Chronic vascular rejection ("allograft vasculopathy," "accelerated atherosclerosis") is characterized by diffuse narrowing of the coronary arteries. These lesions are thought to be secondary to a rejection process and are characterized pathologically by fibrointimal proliferation in a diffuse manner. These lesions do not typically respond to the pharmacologic and surgical interventions used in typical atherosclerosis. This type of rejection can occur in up to as many as 40 percent of patients at three years and is the most common indication for re-transplantation.

Though other protocols are used with equivalent success, many centers employ a three-drug regimen including of cyclosporine, azathioprine, and steroids (Table 29.2).

Given the potency of the three-drug immunosuppressant protocol, patients treated with it are at high risk for infections from bacterial, viral, and fungal pathogens. Any sign of infection is vigorously investigated.

Hypertension develops in 70 to 90 percent of patients following transplantation. The mechanism of hypertension is unknown but is likely related to vasoconstriction, possibly mediated or enhanced by cyclosporine.

Because cyclosporine is a potent nephrotoxic agent, renal insufficiency is common with its use. All of the complications associated with chronic steroid use are also suspect in cardiac transplant patients, including peptic ulcer disease, osteoporosis, and aseptic necrosis of the hip. For this reason, all patients treated with steroids are also given antacids and calcium supplements.

TABLE 29.1 – **Complications of Cardiac Transplantation**

1. Acute rejection
2. Chronic vascular rejection
3. Infection
4. Hypertension
5. Renal insufficiency
6. Obesity
7. Osteoporosis/aseptic necrosis
8. Neoplasia

TABLE 29.2—**University of Minnesota Cardiac Transplant Program**

Immunosuppression Protocol	
Cyclosporine	4 to 6 mg/kg/day (Aim to achieve drug level of 175 ± mg/ml)
Azathioprine	2.0-2.5 mg/kg/day (Titrated to keep WBC greater than 4,000)
Solu-Medrol	500 mg IV on CPB, then 125 mg Q 8H x 24 hours
Prednisone	1.0 mg/kg/day Taper to 10 mg/day by one year

NOTES

#30 References

Antman EM, Smith TW: Pharmacokinetics and digitalis glycosides. In: Digitalis Glycosides. Smith TW (ed.) Orlando: Greene and Stratton, 1985;45.

Arnold SB, et al: Long term digitalis therapy improves left ventricular function in heart failure. N Engl J Med 1980;303:1443.

Baim DS: Effects of amrinone on myocardial energetics in severe congestive heart failure. Am J Cardiol 1985;56:16B-18B.

Braunwald E: Assessment of cardiac function. In: Heart Disease: A Textbook of Cardiovascular Medicine. Braunwald E (ed.) Philadelphia: WB Saunders Co., 1988;449-470.

Braunwald E: Clinical manifestations of heart failure. In: Heart Disease: A Textbook of Cardiovascular Medicine. Braunwald E (ed.) Philadelphia: WB Saunders Co., 1988;471-484.

Braunwald E: Pathophysiology of heart failure. In: Heart Disease: A Textbook of Cardiovascular Medicine. Braunwald E (ed.) Philadelphia: WB Sanders Co., 1988;426-448.

Captopril Multicenter Research Group: A placebo-controlled trial of captopril in refractory chronic congestive heart failure. J Am Coll Cardiol 1983;2:755-763.

Cody RJ, et al: Sodium and water balance in congestive heart failure. J Clin Invest 1986;77:1441.

Cohen DJ et al: Cyclosporine: A new immunosuppressive agent for organ transplantation. Ann Int Med 1984;101:667-682.

Cohn JN, et al: Effect of vasodilator therapy on mortality in chronic congestive heart failure. N Engl J Med 1986;314:1547-1552.

Cohn JN, Franciosa JA: Vasodilator therapy of cardiac failure. N Engl J Med 1977;297:27-31, 254-258.

Colucci WS, et al: New positive inotropic agents in the treatment of congestive heart failure. N Engl J Med 1986;314:290-299, 349-358.

Creager MA, et al: Acute and long-term effects of enalapril in the cardiovascular response to exercise and exercise tolerance in patients with congestive heart failure. J Am Coll Cardiol 1985;6:163.

DiBianco R, et al: Oral milrinone and digoxin in heart failure: Results of a placebo-controlled, prospective trial of each agent and the combination. Abstract. Circ 1987;76:(IV)256.

Doherty JE: Conventional drug therapy in the management of heart failure. In: Drug Treatment of Heart Failure. Cohn JN (ed.) New York: Advanced Therapeutics Communications, Inc., 1983;91-124.

Dzau VJ, et al: Sustained effectiveness of converting enzyme inhibition in patients with severe congestive heart failure. N Engl J Med 1980;302:1373.

Engelmeier RS, et al: Improvement in symptoms and exercise tolerance by metoprolol in patients with dilated cardiomyopathy: A double-blind, randomized, placebo-controlled trial. Circ 1985; 72:536.

Fenoglio JJ, Ursell PC, Kellogg CF: Diagnosis and classification of myocarditis by endomyocardial biopsy. N Engl J Med 1983;308:12-18.

Fowles RE, Mason JW: Endomyocardial biopsy. Ann Int Med 1982;97:885-894.

Francis GS: Inotropic agents in the management of heart failure. In: Drug Treatment of Heart Failure. Cohn JN (ed.) New Jersey: Advanced Therapeutics Communications, Inc., 1988;179-198.

Francis GS, et al: The neurohumoral axis in congestive heart failure. Ann Int Med 1984;101: 370-377.

Goldberg LI, Rajfer SI: Dopamine receptors: Application in clinical cardiology. Circ 1985;72:295-248.

Goldstein S, Pitt B, Captopril Digoxin Multicenter Research Group: Comparative effects of captopril and digoxin in patients with mild to moderate heart failure. JAMA 1988;259:539-544.

Goodwin JF: Cardiac transplantation. Circ 1986; 74:913-916.

Greenburg ML, et al: Long-term hemodynamic follow-up of cardiac transplant patients treated with cyclosporine and prednisone. Circ 1985; 71:487-494.

Hofflin JM, et al: Infectious complications in heart transplant recipients receiving cyclosporine and corticosteroids. Ann Int Med 1987;106:209-216.

Hollenberg NK: Pathophysiology of congestive heart failure: The role of the kidney. In: Drug Treatment of Heart Failure. Cohn JN (ed.) New York: Advanced Therapeutics Communications Inc., 1983;55-72.

Ikram H, et al: Haemodynamic and hormone responses to acute and chronic furosemide therapy in congestive heart failure. Clin Sci Mol Med 1980;59:443.

Johnson RA, Palacios I: Dilated cardiomyopathies of the adult. N Engl J Med 1982;307:1051-1058,1119-1126.

Johnson RA: Heart failure. In: The Practice of Cardiology. Johnson RA, Haber E, Austen WG (eds.) Boston: Little, Brown and Co., 1980;31-95.

Kokko JP: Site and mechanism of action of diuretics. Am J Med 1984;77:11.

Kubo SH, Cody RJ: Clinical and hemodynamic aspects of ACE inhibition for the management of congestive heart failure. In: Angiotensin Converting Enzyme Inhibitors. Ferguson RK, Vlasses PH (eds.) Mount Kisco, NY: Futura Publishing Co., 1987;87-136.

Kubo SH, et al: Identification of normal neurohormonal activity in mild congestive heart failure and the stimulating effect of upright posture and diuretics. Am J Cardiol 1987;60:1322-1329.

Lee DCS, et al: A randomized trial of digoxin versus placebo. N Engl J Med 1982;306:688.

Levine TB, et al: Acute and long-term response to an oral converting enzyme inhibitor, captopril, in congestive heart failure. Circ 1980;62:35.

Marcus FI: Pharmacokinetic interactions between digoxin and other drugs. J Am Coll Cardiol 1985;5:82A.

McKee PA, et al: The natural history of congestive heart failure: The Framingham Study. N Engl J Med 1971;26:1441-1445.

Mikulic E, et al: Comparative hemodynamic effects of inotropic and vasodilator drugs in severe heart failure. Circ 1977;56:528-533.

Miller RR, et al: Combined dopamine and nitroprusside therapy in congestive heart failure: greater augmentation of cardiac performance by addition of inotropic stimulation to afterload reduction. Circ 1977;55:881-884.

Mudge GH, Wainer IM: Drugs affecting renal function and electrolyte metabolism. In: The Pharmacologic Basis of Therapeutics, 7th ed. Gilman AF, et al (eds.) New York: Macmillan, 1985;879-907.

Myers BD, et al: The long-term course of cyclosporine-associated chronic nephropathy. Kid Int 1988;33:590-600.

Packer M: Neurohormonal interactions and adaptations in congestive heart failure. Circ 1988;77:721.

Ross EM, Roberts WC: Severe atherosclerotic coronary artery disease, healed myocardial infarction, and chronic congestive heart failure: Analysis of 81 patients studied at necropsy. Am J Cardiol 1986;57:44-50.

Scholz H: Inotropic drugs and their mechanisms. J Am Coll Cardiol 1984;4:389-397.

Shanes JG, et al: Interobserver variability in the pathologic interpretation of endomyocardial biopsy results. Circ 1987;75:401-405.

Shanes JG: Beta-blockade: Rational or irrational therapy for congestive heart failure. Circ 1987; 76:971-973.

Sharpe DN, et al: Enalapril in patients with chronic heart failure: A placebo-controlled, randomized, double-blind study. Circ 1984;70:271.

Simonton, et al: Milrinone in congestive heart failure: Acute and chronic hemodynamic and clinical evaluation. J Am Coll Cardiol 1985;6:453-459.

Smith TW, et al: The management of heart failure. In: Heart Disease: A Textbook of Cardiovascular Medicine. Braunwald E (ed.) Philadelphia: WB Saunders Co., 1988;485-543.

Sonnenblick EH, et al: Dobutamine: A new synthetic cardioactive sympathetic amine. N Engl J Med 1979;300:17-22.

Swedberg K, et al: Prolongation of survival in congestive cardiomyopathy by beta receptor blockage. Lancet 1979;1:1374.

The CONSENSUS Trial Study Group: Effects of enalapril on mortality in severe congestive heart failure. N Engl J Med 1987;316:1429-1435.

Weber KT, et al: Oxygen utilization and ventilation during exercise in patients with chronic cardiac failure. Circ 1982;65:1213-1223.

Wenger TL, et al: Treatment of 63 severely digitalis toxic patients with digoxin specific antibody fragments. J Am Coll Cardiol 1985;5:118A.

Wynne J, Braunwald E: The cardiomyopathies and myocarditides. In: Heart Disease: A Textbook of Cardiovascular Medicine. Braunwald E (ed.) Philadelphia: WB Saunders Co., 1988;1410-1469.